24-Hour Primary Care

Edited by

Chris Salisbury
Jeremy Dale
and
Lesley Hallam

Radcliffe Medical Press

Radcliffe Medical Press Ltd
18 Marcham Road, Abingdon, Oxon OX14 1AA

British Library Cataloguing in Publication Data

A catalogue record for this book is available from the British Library.

ISBN 1 85775 311 9

Typeset by Advance Typesetting Ltd, Oxfordshire
Printed and bound by Hobbs the Printers, Totton, Hants

Contents

Part Three: Future directions

Preface

Since 1990, a significant reorganisation of primary care services outside normal surgery hours has occurred throughout the UK. This reorganisation has been prompted by an increasing demand from patients for out-of-hours care and an increasing reluctance on the part of general practitioners to spend long and frequent periods on call. However, the UK is not alone among European nations in experiencing these problems and a variety of approaches have been tried both here and in other countries to address these issues. This book describes the antecedents of rising demand and the efforts made or suggested to manage it. The changes in service provision are critically examined, along with the impact of these changes on patients, provider organisations, costs and the health service as a whole. Finally, we examine possible directions for future developments.

A number of themes run throughout the book.

- What is the purpose of out-of-hours care? Is it 'out-of-hours' care or '24-hour' care?
- What are the needs for care? What is the current provision of services and how far does it meet the needs?
- Is demand for care changing? Why is this happening? Can or should demand be managed and if so, how?
- Are the expectations of health professionals changing and if so, why?
- What are the tensions between the expectations of the public and the health professionals? Whose perspectives matter? Are services organised for the benefit of patients or providers?
- What evidence is there about what works? What would make things work better? What are the cost and resource implications?
- How can quality be assured? How should services be monitored?
- How should care be provided? Who should organise it? At what level? Who should pay?

All these questions will be answered in the context of a health service which is undergoing rapid change. Although written from a British perspective, this book also draws on experience from Europe and the United States. It makes a unique contribution to a field which is the source of considerable controversy, but where reliable information and critical analysis of issues are hard to find. Throughout the book we have sought to include quotations (mostly from doctors) which illustrate some of the feelings that these issues have evoked.

The main focus of the book is on care provided by or on behalf of general practitioners, as these are the main providers of out-of-hours services. However, community nurses, ambulance trusts, hospital accident and emergency (A&E) departments, pharmacists and several other professional groups also provide out-of-hours care. The scope for integration of services is another important theme.

The chapters in this book are set out in three sections. The first section describes the background to the recent reorganisation of services, with an analysis of the main dilemmas which have led to the pressure for change. This includes evidence of an increasing disparity between the demands from patients and the expectations of doctors. The section concludes with a framework which describes the various models of organisation for providing out-of-hours general practice care and the claimed advantages of each.

Chapters in the second section describe the main models of organisation in turn. Each chapter considers the underlying factors which determined how and why the model developed as it did, examples of good practice, evidence from evaluations, issues to consider in planning this type of service and suggestions about where the model of care is leading.

The third section considers the future direction of out-of-hours primary care in more detail. Further consideration is given to the importance of assuring quality and the potential for integration of services. Finally, we present a practical vision for the future.

The book will be of interest to all those involved in planning and delivering out-of-hours care. This includes GPs, co-operative and deputising service managers and those involved in commissioning services or forming health policy within primary care organisations, health authorities or at a national level. The book provides a critical overview of the research evidence about the evaluation of out-of-hours services, which will be invaluable to those seeking to evaluate their own organisations, as well as those involved in research or teaching. The issues covered in this book are relevant not only to doctors but also to those involved in planning ambulance services, A&E departments or community nursing services.

The authors combine experience in organising, researching, evaluating and providing out-of-hours care. They come from a range of backgrounds and are well placed to offer practical advice, critical analysis and a political perspective. We hope that this book represents an accessible and useful contribution to the future development of this increasingly important aspect of the health service.

Chris Salisbury
Jeremy Dale
Lesley Hallam
June 1999

List of contributors

Wienke Boerma
Research Fellow
NIVEL Foundation
Netherlands Institute of
    Primary Health Care
PO Box 1568
3500 BN Utrecht
The Netherlands

David Cragg
General Practitioner
250 Park Lane
Macclesfield
Cheshire SK11 8AD

Robert Crouch
Research Fellow & Deputy Director
Centre for the Advancement of
    Clinical Practice
EIHMS
University of Surrey
Guildford
Surrey GU2 5XH

Jeremy Dale
Professor of Primary Health Care
School of Postgraduate Medicine
University of Warwick
Coventry CV4 7AL

Lesley Hallam
Research Fellow
National Primary Care Research &
    Development Centre (NPCRDC)
5th Floor
Williamson Building
University of Manchester
Oxford Road
Manchester M13 9PL

Emma Jefferys
Health Economist
London Health Economics
    Consortium
London School of Hygiene and
    Tropical Medicine
Kepple Street
London WC1E 7HT

Valerie Lattimer
Senior Research Fellow
Health Care Research Unit
University of Southampton
Southampton General Hospital
Level B, South Block
Tremona Road
Southampton SO16 6YD

Robert McKinley
Senior Lecturer in General Practice
Department of General Practice and
   Primary Health Care
University of Leicester
Leicester General Hospital
Gwendolen Road
Leicester LE5 4BP

Mark Reynolds
Chairman
National Association of GP
   Co-operatives
511 Etruria Road
Basford
Stoke on Trent ST4 6HT

Chris Salisbury
Consultant Senior Lecturer
Department of Primary Health Care
University of Bristol
Canynge Hall
Whiteladies Road
Clifton
Bristol BS8 2PR

Cathy Shipman
Research Fellow
Department of Palliative Care &
   Policy
Guy's, King's & St Thomas' School of
   Medicine & Dentistry
Bessemer Road
Denmark Hill
London SE5 9PJ

Alistair Stinson
Clinical Facility Manager/
   Senior Nurse Manager
A&E Department
Central Middlesex Hospital
Acton Lane
Park Royal
London NW10 7NS

PART ONE

Choices and challenges

CHAPTER ONE

Setting the scene

Lesley Hallam

An important feature of any healthcare system is its ability to respond appropriately and quickly when faced with urgent needs for assessment, advice and treatment. From a professional viewpoint, services are required 24 hours a day to diagnose and treat illnesses and injuries which threaten life or limb or carry a high risk of lasting harm without immediate attention. Ambulance services and hospital accident and emergency (A&E) departments operate day and night to meet such needs. Other professional groups, notably those involved in delivering routine primary care, make separate arrangements to meet the emergency needs of their patients at times when they would not normally be accessible. Emergency and out-of-hours services thus overlap, but are not necessarily synonymous. This book concentrates on the particular problems of providing primary medical care out of hours with specific reference to the role of the general practitioner (GP).

Patients frequently lack the knowledge and skills to distinguish between minor illnesses and life-threatening conditions which have symptoms in common. From their viewpoint, 24-hour access to advice, diagnosis and treatment is necessary. Their chosen source of care will reflect the relative accessibility of different services; their perceptions of the different roles of primary and secondary care providers; historical patterns of service utilisation (both within communities and within families); and the costs of accessing services. However, it is clear that thresholds for seeking professional healthcare advice are falling and that this cannot be explained by increased morbidity within populations.

There are obvious and increasing tensions between lay and professional views on access to and appropriate use of emergency services. Demand for primary care services outside normal surgery hours has been rising steadily in the UK for many years.[1,2] Rising demand has been accompanied by an increasing unwillingness among providers, particularly general practitioners, to provide a higher level of service within existing organisational frameworks and remuneration systems.[3] Factors which influence demand and supply are explored in more detail in Chapter Two.

Strategies for managing demand and controlling expenditure are limited. Those which satisfy the needs of funders are unlikely to meet with universal approval from providers and patients. Those which satisfy the needs of providers are unlikely to be acceptable to funders and may be unpopular with patients. Increasingly, the aspirations and behaviour of patients cannot be contained within constraints on human and financial resources.

Introducing measures to control demand is one possible strategy with several elements:

- educating patients in the role and use of emergency services
- reducing the convenience to patients of consulting out of hours
- introducing 'gatekeepers' and barriers to seeking care
- imposing direct patient charges, either universally or in selected instances.

Provider groups and governments have mounted publicity and information campaigns in the past which aimed to educate patients in the 'appropriate' use of services, thus reducing the number of 'unnecessary' out-of-hours calls. There is no measure of their success, but they are widely considered to be ineffective in reaching patients who make frequent use of services for minor problems. There are also fears that they may deter some patients with major problems who would benefit from immediate attention.

The need to ensure that patients can access medical care rapidly in an emergency results in the provision of services which are easily accessible and readily available to all. Consulting a GP in the evening or at weekends may be more convenient to patients than making an appointment to be seen in surgery hours, particularly if the patient can expect to be visited at home. 'Turning up' at an A&E department may be more convenient than first contacting a GP by telephone, especially if A&E departments are geographically closer. To counter this, primary care emergency centres may transfer the onus of travel from the GP to the patient, and patients assigned a low priority by triage nurses in A&E can face lengthy waits for attention at busy periods. Both reduce convenience for patients with minor problems. Unfortunately, they also reinforce the message that although the problem is not urgent, the patient will still be seen.

General practitioners are increasingly choosing to operate telephone triage systems to ensure that only the most urgent cases receive a home visit and the majority of patients must now either travel to a centre or accept telephone advice. In this way, GPs act as their own 'gatekeepers', reducing the number of doctors needed on duty and managing increased levels of demand. However, they are less effective gatekeepers to hospital emergency services. Patients can and do choose to go directly to A&E departments that cannot, by law, turn anyone away.

Imposing direct charges is anathema to many general practitioners. They are not prepared to jeopardise the doctor–patient relationship by introducing a financial element and fear that it would discourage precisely those patients who are likely to be in most need of assistance: the elderly, the socially disadvantaged and children in deprived households. Nonetheless, it has been argued that charges would dramatically reduce the number of non-essential out-of-hours consultations. A&E departments can make a charge for their services but only when the patient is a road traffic accident victim and might reasonably be expected to make an insurance claim covering the cost of treating injuries.

Although the manner in which European health services have chosen to define, organise and fund emergency care varies from country to country, the UK is not alone in facing problems in providing out-of-hours care. There have been increasing tensions between policymakers and medical care providers relating to the organisation, staffing and funding of emergency services in many other countries. As demand rises, governments and third-party payers who meet the costs of care seek to control expenditure. Healthcare professionals seek greater financial rewards and reductions in their workload.[4,5]

This chapter sets out some of the main themes and dilemmas in out-of-hours care which are common internationally.

The role of general practitioners

In the UK, general practitioners are personally responsible for ensuring that their registered patients have access to primary medical care 24 hours a day, seven days a week. Until recently, this has normally meant that patients calling out of hours have been visited in their homes, either by a GP from their own practice working in a rota or by a commercial deputising service acting on behalf of the practice.[6] Under normal circumstances, GPs act as gatekeepers to expensive, hospital-based services. However, in an emergency, and particularly out of hours, patients can independently choose to attend a hospital A&E department and may summon an ambulance to take them there. In larger population centres, they may also be able to seek advice from 24-hour pharmacies. Other professional groups also provide 24-hour cover – for instance, community nurses, mental health teams and dentists. However, it is the GP who is at the heart of the UK system.

The central role of individual GPs is not unique in European healthcare systems, but it is becoming increasingly rare to find systems which closely mirror our own. The Netherlands is generally acknowledged to be the most similar. There, GPs continue to provide the majority of out-of-hours emergency care through rota systems, visiting patients in their homes. There is direct access to hospital first aid departments and many patients choose this route into care. Similarities between the UK and The Netherlands have given rise to similar problems: demand is rising, patients complain of limited access to services and Dutch GPs complain of increasing workloads, stress and 'burnout'.

In recent years, British GPs have increasingly chosen to form and join out-of-hours co-operatives, providing emergency cover for the patients of all member practices. They ask patients to attend an emergency centre, visiting patients at home only when it is considered medically necessary (*see* Chapter Five). Denmark instituted a similar system in 1992, but on a nationwide rather than an *ad hoc* basis. Two of the principal reasons for the Danish reforms were growing demand (particularly from young people) and pressure from young doctors for greater income and lower workload. Denmark's central facilities theoretically act as gatekeepers to secondary care in all but the most serious cases. However, this has not prevented patients using hospital A&E departments to answer their primary care needs, either because it is more convenient or because they are dissatisfied with the attention they receive from the primary care facilities, which rely heavily on telephone advice.

There are also lessons to be learned from the system which operates in Finland. Finland, in common with the UK and The Netherlands, relies heavily upon general practitioners. Many large health centres are required by local regulation to stay open throughout the night and patients of these and neighbouring, smaller health centres are advised to go there first. In theory, only serious accidents, life-threatening acute conditions and acute obstetric needs are treated in specialist hospital facilities without professional referral. In rural areas, ambulances are encouraged to transport patients first to a local health centre. As a result, health centre waiting rooms are crowded throughout the evenings and weekends, with patients using the out-of-hours service as a convenient alternative to daytime consulting. Since opening is mandatory, there is little incentive to organise daytime services more efficiently to reduce out-of-hours workload. In recent years some health centres have been allowed to commission services from a local specialist hospital to provide cover at times when demand would normally be very low. This has simply raised fears that the principle of 'primary care first' is being eroded.

Pressure for change in the role of GPs in providing out-of-hours care was intense in Britain in the early 1990s. The majority of GPs believed that there should be provision to opt out of 24-hour responsibilities for those who wished to do so. There was some support for the introduction of a split contract, in which normal surgery responsibilities and out-of-hours responsibilities would be separately costed and GPs would have the freedom to accept the contract of their choice. Growing numbers of part-time GPs, female GPs and salaried GPs, many of whom were not playing a full part in out-of-hours rotas, reinforced calls for reform. Given that many GPs would choose to provide daytime services only and given that fewer medical graduates are currently entering British general practice, this could have led to chaos. As well as insufficient medical manpower to support such a split service, a number of other disadvantages of a split service have been described.

- It might undermine the concept of the 'family doctor' which is at the heart of the primary care system.
- There is a danger that the out-of-hours service would be second-rate, with lower status and less competent doctors.
- There is a risk that the two services would be unco-ordinated, creating communication gaps in patient care.

However, it could be argued that the above problems may also occur with any out-of-hours services organised outside an individual practice, such as deputising services and co-operatives, whether or not the out-of-hours service is formally separated from the daytime service.

In the UK, the government is committed to maintaining 24-hour responsibility for patient care within the system of patient registration with an individual practice. In this, they are supported by most elements of the medical profession, along with health authorities, ambulance trusts and some A&E staff. They believe that the future of out-of-hours care in the UK lies in greater co-ordination and co-operation between existing services.

A number of European systems can offer examples of where moves away from a 24-hour contract might lead.

In Sweden, 95% of general practitioners are employed by their county council and work 40 hours a week by law. They rely on a combination of primary healthcare centres in urban areas, which rarely open throughout the night, and small rotas of local GPs in rural areas. Night-time care is often available only in hospitals, where GPs may be employed to triage and treat patients. Sweden has relied historically on hospital services and despite increasing emphasis on the role of primary care, a high proportion of patients choose to attend A&E departments, regardless of the higher direct charges associated with this. The limitation on general practitioners' hours of work results in poorer access to daytime services for patients, since doctors are frequently off duty in compensation for hours worked outside the normal surgery day.

General practitioners in Portugal are also salaried employees of their national health service and are thus required to provide out-of-hours care as part of their contractual responsibilities. These services are provided at central facilities, though there are also small groups of private providers who undertake domiciliary visits for a fee. Whilst patients can access hospital services directly, there is an additional fee for this. Demand for evening and weekend consultations has increased the number of GPs needed on duty at 'unsocial' hours, with consequent reductions in daytime access to services and increased salary costs for the health service. There are also problems in co-ordinating daytime and out-of-hours care.

Throughout the European Union, the introduction of restrictions on the number of hours that employees can be required to work will have important implications for salaried health services.

In Italy, GPs are not on duty during evenings, nights, weekends and major holidays. There is a parallel service out of hours, called Medical Guard, which is nationwide and accessed by a toll-free telephone number. This service provides home visits and advice or hospitalisation. It cannot organise specialist referrals, except emergency hospital admissions, and has a number of other limitations imposed upon it. There are considerable problems in communication between daytime and out-of-hours services. Whilst patients can go directly to hospital emergency rooms, they may be charged for services if their case is not judged to be urgent by the hospital doctors. The system is extremely expensive and there are moves afoot to abolish Medical Guard and place the responsibility for first-contact emergency care with GPs to reduce costs.

Other countries are also trying to increase the involvement of GPs in providing an out-of-hours service, largely because alternative systems have proved very much more expensive. Spain is in the process of reforming its system. Patients have historically relied on hospital emergency services, due to poor access and poor quality in primary care. In many towns, large rotas of general practitioners operating from primary care centres are becoming more common, where attempts are made to screen callers and direct them to the most appropriate source of care. Outside major population centres, the situation is less clearcut. Attitudes are proving slow to change and further reforms are planned, including the imposition of direct charges for patients attending hospital facilities with primary care problems.

The role of different provider groups

Although the GPs' role is central to the UK system and they are the first point of contact for the majority of out-of-hours callers, a wide range of other health services also provide emergency cover on a 24-hour basis. Chief among these are the hospital-based emergency services including major trauma centres, A&E departments and minor injury units staffed by GPs, clinical assistants, hospital doctors or, increasingly, nurse practitioners. One of the greatest stumbling blocks to integrating services is resistance on the part of many A&E departments to anything which might open their doors to more primary care cases. Patients can choose to access these services directly rather than make initial contact with their GP and many do so in circumstances which are considered inappropriate.[7-9]

As has already been shown, the UK is not alone in experiencing difficulties drawing a dividing line between A&E services and primary care services and persuading patients to accept that division. The Netherlands, Denmark and Sweden also have this problem.

In France, whilst doctors are obliged to provide 24-hour care and most are in rotas with colleagues or deputising doctors, more patients are handled by four other services: a public '999' service attached to hospitals (SAMU); a private organisation of night and weekend doctors (SOS Medecins); direct access to hospital A&E services; and access to first aid and ambulance facilities provided by fire services. Whilst this results in an abundant supply of services and a high degree of patient choice, the overlap between services is both expensive and inefficient. There is little co-ordination between the various provider groups.

Germany and Norway have chosen a somewhat different approach to the problem of providing adequate access to out-of-hours emergency care. In Germany, all office-based physicians in the ambulatory care sector are required to play an equal part in providing emergency out-of-hours cover. Patients are not registered with general practitioners and are not expected to call their own GP first in the event of a problem. The physicians on duty out of hours are not necessarily GPs or internists. They may equally well specialise in particular branches of medicine, for instance paediatrics and gastro-enterology. There are clear distinctions between the medical rescue services and the emergency out-of-hours service provided as a standard benefit of statutory health insurance. In many areas there is competition between regularly organised services and private providers.

Norway has a similar system. Traditional practice/health centre rotas have been replaced by large rotas organised at local government level that include hospital- and university-based physicians. They operate a combined centre-based and home visiting service, but general practitioners try to limit their participation in these rotas, which again introduces problems in providing acceptable and appropriate care.

There remain a number of other countries in which A&E departments are the principal source of primary out-of-hours care and this is an accepted feature of their service. Greece, for instance, operates a system which is almost entirely hospital based, with no properly developed system of general practitioner care, except in some rural health centres. Direct visits to the emergency rooms of various hospital centres are the norm.

Clearly, there are considerable differences in the organisation of out-of-hours, emergency services throughout Europe and within individual countries. Equally clearly, they share similar problems:

- defining the role of different provider groups
- ensuring the appropriate provision and utilisation of services

- apportioning responsibility for organisation and management
- improving co-ordination and communication between services
- controlling costs.

What is appropriate care?

Healthcare provider groups view much of their out-of-hours workload as 'inappropriate' in that it does not constitute what they would define as medical emergencies. British general practitioners claim that a high proportion of their calls relate to minor, self-limiting conditions which do not require immediate treatment. Estimates of the proportion of calls which constitute genuine emergencies or at least a necessary call for medical assistance vary from 30% to 60%, dependent upon the definition applied and the personal judgement of the GPs involved.[1,10,11,12]

A&E departments are organised to meet the needs of patients with major trauma or life-threatening illness. They too complain that they are treating 'inappropriate' attenders. In the UK, A&E departments suggest that most of their inappropriate attenders could have been seen by general practitioners. Again, estimates of the proportion of attendances involved vary between 5% and 80%, dependent upon the definition applied and the personal judgement of the staff involved.[1,8,9,13,14] Triage systems operate to 'stream' primary care and hospital A&E patients and to ensure that the most urgent cases are seen rapidly, but patients with problems judged to be non-urgent often face lengthy waits for attention. Nevertheless, attendances at most A&E departments are rising year-on-year.

Whilst patients' actions may be seen as 'inappropriate' from a provider viewpoint, from a consumer viewpoint it is the services which are inappropriately organised and structured to meet their needs. At present, there is limited emphasis on matching services to the needs and wishes of patients. Rather, services are configured to reflect professional values, medically defined needs and available resources, both financial and human.

One initiative designed to address the needs of patients with primary care problems who choose to attend an A&E department is reported in Chapter Six. A&E departments have employed general practitioners on a sessional basis to handle primary care patients. Despite evidence of its success and cost-effectiveness, it has not been widely adopted. A directly opposing philosophy involves greater separation and stratification of services. Regional trauma centres will take the most serious cases from acute hospital A&E departments. Minor accident units, often nurse led with GP and hospital doctor back-up, will take the least serious cases. As a result, fewer general A&E departments will be needed and hence fewer will be available to treat patients with conditions which are not considered medically 'appropriate' to an A&E environment.

There is much debate about the wider role that nurses could play in providing services outside normal surgery hours. In the UK, community nurses already respond to emergency situations at the behest of GPs and patients who are already on their routine care lists, as well as offering pre-planned 24-hour care. However, it has been suggested that nurses could be employed more widely in primary care emergency centres to triage telephone calls and provide advice and treatment to patients with minor injuries and illnesses (*see* Chapter Seven).

In its favour, nursing input would reduce the workload of on-call general practitioners, relieving them of callers who do not need the skill levels of GPs to solve their problems. However, there are a wide range of obstacles to their greater deployment.

- Nurses are expensive, especially in comparison with GPs who are relatively poorly rewarded for their out-of-hours responsibilities.
- Whilst nurses would reduce GP workload, they would not necessarily reduce their rota commitments, particularly in small rotas where the same limited number of GPs would still have to be on duty alongside nursing staff.
- Many GPs would be unhappy with nurse triage, believing GPs to be 'safer', more effective and more flexible in that role.
- Current legislation holds GPs legally responsible in any cases of mismanagement of their registered patients by their agents.
- There are insufficient numbers of appropriately trained nurses to meet potential demand and the nursing profession is itself facing a recruitment and retention problem.

A recent initiative promoted by the Department of Health is NHS Direct, a separate 24-hour telephone advice service for patients seeking information on self-care or direction to the most appropriate source of professional help. The service is staffed by trained nurses. It has the potential to take over a gatekeeper role from general practitioners, channelling patients to general practitioner, hospital, ambulance and other health services, though this is not currently part of its remit.

It has also been suggested that paramedics could make a significant contribution to the primary care out-of-hours workforce. However, paramedics are currently trained in a limited number of specialist skills, for instance resuscitation and stabilisation in cases of major illness and trauma. Such cases are not representative of GPs' out-of-hours workload. A new cadre of 'care assistants' with limited triage and treatment skills might be more appropriate, but would take time to establish and would probably meet with considerable resistance from the nursing professions.

The involvement of the full primary care team in 24-hour care, so that GPs, practice nurses, community nurses and a variety of other professionals allied to medicine would be available to provide appropriate advice and treatment for patients, implies an acceptance that the service is moving from out-of-hours emergency cover to 24-hour access to primary care. Whilst many GPs believe that patients already treat the service in this way, there would be strong opposition to any developments which reinforced this view.

Organisation structures for general practitioners

In the UK, at whatever level of aggregation general practitioners choose to provide an emergency primary care service (individually, in a practice rota or in a co-operative rota), it is they who are responsible for its organisation. Only by employing a commercial deputising service, at considerable personal expense, can they delegate organisational matters. General practitioners in Belgium and The Netherlands are likewise responsible for organising their own services.

However, in Denmark, planning and administrative responsibility is shared between doctors' regional associations and local government. In Sweden, county councils have full responsibility for organising out-of-hours care. In Germany, much of the organisation falls to regional physicians' associations rather than individual GPs. In Italy, a totally separate, government-organised service looks after patients' needs outside normal surgery hours.

There is a case to be made in the UK for the creation of some form of umbrella organisations which would provide centralised communications and triage systems and undertake administrative and management functions on behalf of groups of GPs affiliated to them. The growing number of GP co-operatives (described in Chapter Five) is evidence of the feasibility of this approach but it is as yet piecemeal and co-operatives vary widely in their size, sophistication and degree of centralisation. Health authorities, who hold the contracts of all general practitioners working in their area, might have taken this responsibility before the introduction of the 'internal' market in the NHS. However, their role is now limited to commissioning rather than providing health services and they are therefore unlikely candidates for this additional responsibility.

A new development in primary care involves the formation of primary care groups (PCGs). These groups include all GPs in a defined area, covering 'natural' communities and population groups of around 100 000 patients and thus containing approximately 60 GPs. They incorporate community nursing services, and are expected to work in partnership with other agencies providing health and social care to improve the health of their local population.

It is intended that they will jointly commission secondary care and other medical services; maintain financial control of their own budgets; monitor the performance of the secondary and ancillary care services which they purchase; monitor and improve the performance of member practices and integrate primary, community and social services. With this very broad remit, they could well serve as umbrella organisations for their members' out-of-hours services, though this might well cut across the boundaries of existing out-of-hours care groups.

Funding and costs

In the majority of European countries, patients face some financial penalty for seeing a GP out of hours (though this may be only a little higher than the payment they would also make for care during normal surgery hours). Either they are asked to pay the general practitioner the full fee directly (part of which may be reclaimed from their insurer) or they are asked to make an immediate co-payment, with the remainder being paid by their insurer. Denmark and Great Britain are notable exceptions to this system, with virtually all patients receiving care free at the point of delivery. Throughout Europe, charges are also commonly made for treatment in A&E departments. Such charges are often used to influence patients' behaviour. For instance, hospital fees may be higher than GP fees and may be increased in cases where attendance is considered inappropriate.

Payment systems for general practitioners are extremely complex, ranging from 'overtime' payments and time off in lieu for those who are salaried, through systems of capitation fees and allowances, to fees for services rendered, with some systems incorporating various elements into hybrid systems. Paymasters will include patients, insurance companies, mutual funds and government departments. Clearly, the way in which payments are calculated and the total amount which general practitioners receive for their on-call work have a considerable influence upon their working patterns and their attitudes towards out-of-hours work.

For example, Spanish GPs in rural areas are predominantly independent contractors. They receive capitation fees and a small additional allowance to reflect the fact that they may be called upon outside normal surgery hours. There is little incentive to offer a 24-hour service. In contrast, Finnish GPs receive a fee for service outside office hours, which has promoted their willingness to provide out-of-hours services at the expense of office hours services which do not attract such a fee. The Danish system also incorporates a scale of fees for services, which has been skewed to encourage telephone advice at the expense of surgery attendances and home visits. As a result, the pattern of care provided has changed but with the unwanted side-effect of increasing the attractions of A&E attendance for patients dissatisfied with the advice they receive.

In the UK, each GP currently receives an allowance of £2245 per annum (January 1999) from the National Health Service to reflect his or her responsibility for providing 24-hour care. There is also a fee of around £22 for each patient seen between 10.00 pm and 8.00 am. No fees are payable for patients seen during evenings and weekend days. With an average list size and average demand for out-of-hours care, this represents approximately £3300 in income. There is also a development fund with an annual budget of £45 million to support and underwrite GP-led initiatives to improve the organisation and quality of out-of-hours care. Principally, this has been used to develop and support co-operatives (*see* Chapter Five). Although this sum equates to approximately £1400 per annum for each GP, it represents only a partial subsidy for the costs of the infrastructure needed to provide out-of-hours services and cannot be used to pay GPs.

General practitioners argue that this level of remuneration is poor reward for the number of hours they spend on call and the work which they actually do. Since they are responsible for providing the infrastructure to offer 24-hour services, they argue that it should not be necessary to sacrifice a portion of this income to fund a more efficient service.

'I've worked out [that] if you average out the amount of money you get over the year and what you have to cover for, you actually get paid more for being a baby-sitter than you do for being a GP paid by the government to provide 24-hour emergency medical care to your patients.'

'We are paying to go to work. Do you know anybody else who does that?'

(Interview transcripts, case studies of GP co-operatives, to be published.)

The heavy reliance on hospital-based services evident in some European systems is said to result in considerably more expensive services. It is difficult to assess the precise impact of this. Emergency departments need to be equipped with expensive, specialised equipment and to have specially trained staff available 24 hours a day. Reducing the number of primary care patients attending could reduce staff costs, but will have little impact on the costs of providing equipment and infrastructure. Primary care patients represent a marginal increase in cost, rather than a *pro rata* cost. Nonetheless, many countries are trying to move to systems which promote the role of the general practitioner, particularly as a gatekeeper, in order to cut costs. To do this, they must strengthen the infrastructure and organisation of general practice and offer sufficiently attractive remuneration to general practitioners to bring them willingly into a new system. The costs of this have not been quantified and given the growing resistance to 24-hour responsibility among general practitioners who currently hold it, changing from a hospital-based culture of emergency care may not be easily or cheaply accomplished.

Conclusion

Throughout much of Europe, rising demand, rising costs, poorly co-ordinated services and provider dissatisfaction with workload and remuneration are prompting debate on how current systems of out-of-hours care can be reformed to produce more cost-effective, efficient services which answer patients' needs.

There are three fundamental political questions which need to be addressed before any further attempts are made to reform the current system of out-of-hours care in the UK.

- Whose interests are paramount: government, providers or patients?
- Should the system provide only emergency primary care or 24-hour access to routine primary care?
- Should the service be the responsibility of individual providers and provider groups or a broader regional or national responsibility?

A 24-hour access service, run to serve the interests and preferences of patients, with the responsibility resting on individual providers is a very different organisation from a regionally funded and managed emergency service which balances costs with the interests of professionals and patients. Out-of-hours care has been moving very much in the direction of the former until recently, but with no official recognition of this fact. GPs themselves are trying to move the responsibility from individuals to groups, reasserting the need to balance professional and patient interests and attempting to stem non-emergency use of the service by decreasing its convenience to patients.

Succeeding chapters document changes in demand and supply and the factors which influence them, examine different models of primary care outside normal surgery hours and discuss possible future directions.

References

1   Hallam L (1994) Primary medical care outside normal working hours: review of published work. *BMJ*. **308**: 249–53.

2   Doctors and Dentists Review Body (1991) *General Medical Practitioners' Workload Survey 1989–90*. Department of Health, London.

3   Electoral Reform Ballot Services (1992) *Your Choices for the Future: a survey of GP opinion, UK report*. ERBS, London.

4   Sheldon T, Roberts J, Dorozynski A *et al.* (1994) Out of hours care – a round up. *BMJ*. **308**: 1388–91.

5   Frijns MM (1997) *Acute Health Care Out of Hours. Primary care solutions in Denmark, Sweden, the United Kingdom, Belgium and the Netherlands examined.* Maastricht University and NIVEL, Utrecht.

6   Hallam L, Cragg D (1994) Organisation of primary care services outside normal working hours. *BMJ.* **309**: 1621–23.

7   Cohen J (1987) Accident and emergency services and general practice – conflict or co-operation? *Family Pract.* **4**: 81–3.

8   Prince A, Worth CA (1992) A study of 'inappropriate' attendances to a paediatric accident and emergency department. *J Publ Health Med.* **14**: 177–82.

9   Shipman C, Longhurst S, Hollenbach F, Dale J (1997) Using out of hours services: general practice or A&E? *Family Pract.* **14**: 503–9.

10 Tulloch AJ (1984) 'Out-of-hours' calls in an Oxfordshire practice. *Practitioner.* **228**: 663–6.

11 Riddell JA (1980) Out-of-hours visits in a group practice. *BMJ.* **ii**: 1518–19.

12 Dale J, Green J, Reid F, Glucksman E (1995) Primary care in the accident and emergency department: I. Prospective identification of patients. *BMJ.* **311**: 423–6.

13 Green J, Dale J (1992) Primary care in accident and emergency and general practice: a comparison. *Soc Sci Med.* **35**: 987–95.

14 Driscoll PA, Vincent CA, Wilkinson M (1987) The use of the accident and emergency department. *Arch Emerg Med.* **4**: 77–82.

CHAPTER TWO

Balancing demand and supply in out-of-hours care

Chris Salisbury and Wienke Boerma

In order to plan an effective out-of-hours primary care service it is necessary to organise a level of supply of services which balances the demand for that service from patients. In fact, as we shall see later, supply and demand for healthcare are not independent, but are inextricably linked. The level of demand is strongly related to the level of supply. When they are in balance the service is likely to run smoothly. Many aspects of health services operate under a constant tension with demand always exceeding supply, as exemplified by the perennial problem of waiting lists for operations. Improvements in the provision of services lead to greater demand, as more people seek to benefit from care. This problem is particularly acute in the context of out-of-hours primary care. As we discussed in the previous chapter, there has been a growing mismatch between an increasing demand from patients for out-of-hours services and a decreasing willingness from GPs to work at unsocial hours. This has led to pressures for change in the system. This chapter provides a more detailed understanding of the changing level of demand and of the factors which have influenced doctors' willingness to supply services.

What is the demand for out-of-hours care?

Accurate information about the demand for care is an essential prerequisite for the planning of appropriate services. However, the necessary information is not readily available from any one source and the data that are available have often been collected in small local areas and may be of limited applicability elsewhere. This chapter seeks to draw together the results from a number of different studies, to provide essential guidance for those discussing new developments in out-of-hours care. Information is needed about the following.

- Who calls? Which groups of patients are most likely to request out-of-hours care?
- Why do they call? What are the most common problems about which people consult? What are the background factors which lead to a call and what do we know about the types of help that people are seeking?
- When do people call? What is the pattern of consultations, what are the times of peak demand and how does demand vary by day of the week or month of the year?
- Which services do people call? General practitioners are one part of a network which includes ambulance services, A&E departments and community nurses. What proportion of out-of-hours care is provided by these different agencies?
- How many people call and how does this vary in different settings?

What do we mean by 'demand'?

The concept of 'demand' needs clarification. The plain English idea of demand suggests the notion of a request or a perceived need. In considering health services, demand for care has often been equated with the level of activity of a service. However, this assumes that a patient's perceived need always results in a contact with the health service. This ignores the possibility that people may wish to contact a doctor outside surgery hours, but are unable to do so because of a lack of knowledge about how to make contact, communication and language difficulties or the lack of availability of a telephone. These problems may be widespread, particularly in inner-city areas. Apparent increases in demand may simply reflect increased accessibility, for example as more people have telephones in their homes. The level of expressed demand from patients is also related to their expectations of the service. People may feel they need help but not bother to contact a service if they feel that help will not be available.

Although the above points should be remembered, the only readily available information about demand for out-of-hours care is based on the recorded levels of activity of primary care services. This information is difficult to interpret because different organisations have collected different types of data. The reliability of the data, the definitions used and the time periods studied have all varied. It is also apparent that there is a striking variation in demand in different settings and in different parts of the country, making it difficult to generalise or predict the demand for out-of-hours primary care in a particular situation.

Who calls?

In planning out-of-hours service, it is important to note that certain patient groups generate a large proportion of the primary care workload in the out-of-hours period. In particular, calls from parents about children aged less than five years account for up to a quarter of all out-of-hours calls.[1] These calls about young children are most frequent in the evening. Overall call rates are lower for older children and teenagers and then steadily rise with increasing age (Figure 2.1). Areas which contain a large number of young children may therefore expect a higher number of out-of-hours calls, although this may be counterbalanced by the high proportion of young adults in such areas, who tend to call infrequently.

Women are much more likely to call outside normal surgery hours than men, although it appears that calls about infants more often concern boys than girls. The difference in call rates is greatest during the reproductive years. This pattern of consultation rates in different age-sex groups is similar to that seen in daytime general practice.

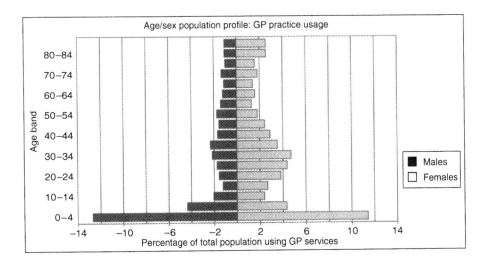

Figure 2.1:   Contact rates by age and sex[2]

Why do people call?

A relatively small number of different problems account for a large proportion of the calls to out-of-hours services. In view of the frequency of calls about young children, the problems on this list are unsurprising. The most common problems presented to out-of-hours primary care services are:

- respiratory tract infections
- diarrhoea and vomiting
- children with earache
- children with a temperature
- minor injuries.

The question about why people call can, however, be addressed in a different way. There is a considerable body of literature about the factors which trigger a consultation with the doctor in the daytime. It is well recognised that one must consider the context to the problem and, in particular, the ideas and expectations of the patient with regard to their symptoms. Less attention has been given to these issues with regard to out-of-hours consultations.

Interviews with people after they have contacted a doctor in the evening suggest that their concern about the importance of particular symptoms (particularly the threat of meningitis), their previous experience of making out-of-hours calls and their need to gain a sense of control in a frightening situation are all important factors which lead to an out-of-hours call.[3,4] The severity, duration and acuteness of the complaint also help to determine whether a person seeks healthcare.[5] All these findings confirm that issues prompting patients' help-seeking behaviour outside normal surgery hours are similar to those that affect daytime consulting. The pursuit of a model of out-of-hours care based on medical necessity that neglects the psychosocial context of illness may not be appropriate.[4]

When do people call?

The peak levels of demand for out-of-hours care follow a fairly consistent pattern. Call rates are highest in the early evening and then tail off between 10.00 pm and 1.00 am. The number of calls between 1.00 am and 6.00 am is low, but rises between 6.00 am and 8.00 am (Figure 2.2). Call rates appear to be higher on weekend nights than on weekdays, although this finding is not consistently reported. For organisations such as co-operatives and deputising services, the time of peak demand is Sunday morning, with calls becoming less frequent in the afternoons. It is likely that more calls are made in the

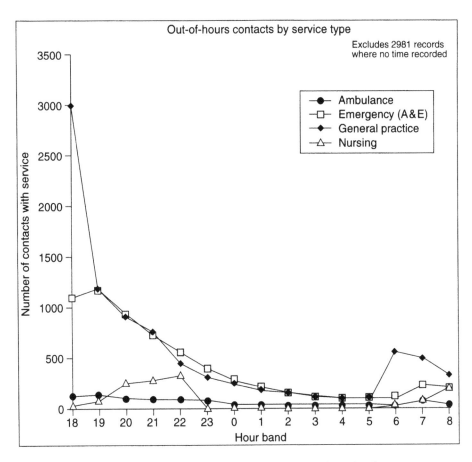

Figure 2.2: Times of calls to out-of-hours services in Buckinghamshire[2]

winter than in the summer, although reports on this issue are surprisingly contradictory and there is little robust evidence available.

Who do people call?

It is interesting to consider the proportion of care which is provided by general practice, in relation to the demands made on other services. One factor which will influence the rate of out-of-hours calls made to general practitioners is the range of alternative sources of help available to patients. Primary care is provided not only by GPs but also by A&E departments, ambulance services, pharmacists and community nurses. However, GPs appear to be the main providers of out-of-hours primary care, providing about half of all contacts, with A&E departments providing a further third of contacts.[6,7] This balance is related both to the age of the patient needing attention and to the time of day or night. Calls about young children are more commonly made to GPs, but young adults are more likely to attend the local A&E department. In the early hours of the morning most calls are made to A&E, but during the day at weekends most callers contact their GPs.[8]

As with the overall level of demand, these findings may vary considerably in different settings. An important factor affecting where people attend for out-of-hours care may be the proximity and accessibility of A&E departments. There may also be differences between urban and rural areas. London in particular has a different tradition, with many people using A&E departments to meet their needs for primary care. General practitioners in London appear to carry out low numbers of out-of-hours calls. This is an important finding for the planning of health services, as it is in marked contrast to other metropolitan areas where call rates tend to be high.

How many people call? The variation in demand

An average GP co-operative might expect to receive between 140 and 240 out-of-hours calls (between 7.00 pm and 7.00 am or at weekends after midday on Saturday) per 1000 patients per annum. However, there is considerable variation in the numbers of out-of-hours calls reported from different parts of the country, between different local areas and even between different practices working from the same health centre.

What might be the reasons for this variation? In answering this question, we need to consider both characteristics of the patients and the local area ('demand factors') and issues related to the provision of services ('supply factors').

The balance of supply and demand
Demand factors

We have already seen that age and sex are related to rates of out-of-hours calls; therefore the demographic characteristics of local populations are likely to influence the demand on health services. We have also discussed the importance of understanding patients' health beliefs in determining whether an illness results in a call for professional help or whether it is managed at home. These beliefs are partly reflections of cultural values which may vary between and within different countries.

One approach to understanding the variation in demand is to relate out-of-hours attendance rates to characteristics of geographical areas. It has been found that out-of-hours call rates are strongly related to the levels of material deprivation of an area, indicated by areas with high levels of unemployment, overcrowded housing, low levels of car ownership and low rates of owner occupation.[7] Areas with high levels of illness, evidenced by high standardised mortality rates and high numbers of patients reporting chronic illness, not surprisingly generate high numbers of out-of-hours calls.[9]

Supply-related factors

Factors related to supply can be subdivided into those that relate to the national healthcare system (organisation and financing) and those related to the local situation (access, practice conditions and organisation of duty arrangements).

Features of the healthcare system can influence the use that is made of acute healthcare out of hours. An important aspect of the organisation of the healthcare system in this respect is 'gatekeeping' by general practitioners. The notion that effective primary care reduces patient usage of A&E departments is widely accepted. Gatekeeping by GPs is a central feature of healthcare in several countries in Europe, such as the United Kingdom and The Netherlands. The contractual obligation to provide 24-hour care to patients on a GP's list helps to reduce unnecessary use of A&E departments. In a study in France, the lack of a gatekeeping general practitioner was found to be a major risk factor for non-urgent visits to an A&E department.[10] It appears to be increasingly common, particularly in big cities, for patients to use A&E departments for non-urgent acute pathology that could have been dealt with by the general practitioner. Patients then reach a more specialised medical echelon which is less efficient, more expensive and damaging to the continuity of care.

The financing of healthcare is also relevant. It has frequently been suggested that if patients paid directly for out-of-hours care, this would reduce unnecessary calls. The contradictory argument is that charges would have the greatest deterrent effect on the poorest members of a community, who are likely to have the greatest needs for care.

There are two ways in which doctors can be paid: either by direct payment (by government, a sickness fund or insurer) or by the patient (who may be reimbursed for it). In the latter case, there are three possibilities:

- co-insurance: the patient has to pay a percentage of the costs of care
- co-payments: the patient pays a fixed amount of money per item of service
- deductible: the patient pays all the costs up to a ceiling.

The effects of co-payments have been studied in health maintainance organisations (HMOs) in the United States. In one study, the introduction of a small co-payment for the use of the emergency department was associated with a decline of about 15% in the use of that department, mostly among patients with conditions considered likely not to present an emergency.[11] In another study, based on data from the Rand Health Insurance Experiment, patients liable for co-payments were significantly less likely to visit the emergency department in the following three years.[12] The absolute size of the co-payment did not seem to be of influence and the effect of co-payments applied similarly to both urgent and less urgent diagnoses. For accidents or serious illness, the co-payments had no effect. Reductions in the appropriate use of services where even brief delays may be harmful and produce adverse effects on health were not demonstrated. It is important to note that the above studies were conducted in the United States; it cannot be assumed that the same findings would be made in countries with different traditions of healthcare.

The way in which physicians are paid is thought to affect physicians' behaviour and the outcome of this behaviour in turn affects healthcare utilisation and costs. This effect can be demonstrated by considering the payment systems in different European countries. The remuneration systems differ with respect to the relation between income, on the one hand, and time invested in providing care, on the other. In a fee-for-service system, a GP is rewarded for the investment of extra time, whereas the opposite occurs under a capitation payment system. Fee-for-service systems are well recognised to induce more activity. The impact of these differences is evident in the provision of out-of-hours primary care.[13]

In Denmark, for example, the fee-for-service system gave rise to ever-increasing costs for the night service. In 1990, out-of-hours services were reformed in Denmark. General practitioners continued to be paid on a fee-for-service basis, but different fees were set according to the type of care provided. Danish GPs receiving patients' out-of-hours telephone calls were given an incentive to complete calls by offering telephone advice alone, since the fee for this was higher than for offering patients a clinic consultation or home visit. Home visits were paid according to the time taken to complete a visit. Following the reforms, the proportion of calls handled on the telephone increased considerably.[14] In the UK, the effects of changes in the payment structure for night visits can also be seen. In 1990, the period during which general practitioners could claim night visit fees was extended by two hours and a differential payment was introduced with a higher rate for visits made by the GP personally and a lower rate for visits made by doctors from a deputising service. The number of night visits rose, which could not be completely attributed to the extended hours for which GPs could claim night visits, while the proportion of visits carried out by deputies fell by more than half.[1]

The organisation of general practice and of A&E departments at the local level varies in terms of accessibility, practice conditions and organisation of duty arrangements. Roberts and Mays[15] reviewed the literature on this subject and concluded that improved access to primary care where access was previously poor could reduce emergency department utilisation. Lack of access to a GP appears to be one of the major determinants of attending an A&E department[5] and the association between A&E attendance and distance has been shown in several studies, mostly set in rural areas.

An effective system of general practice requires an optimal level of accessibility and availability of services. These principles have consequences for the organisation of the practice. In fact, there are several barriers to seeking primary care, whether routinely or in a perceived emergency. These include difficulties in obtaining an appointment, problems in travelling and waiting times in the surgery.

There has been a suggestion that the use of deputising services increases the number of out-of-hours calls, but the evidence for this is doubtful.[9,16] Other features of practice organisation may be more important. In one study, there was a twofold difference in the number of night visits conducted by practices operating from the health centre and covering the same geographical area.[17] This finding, which is consistent with other research, suggests that factors within general practices lead to variation in out-of-hours call rates, which cannot fully be accounted for by differences in the characteristics of the population or the area. Although practice factors appear to be important, the exact nature of these factors is so far unexplained. There is no clear evidence that aspects of primary care organisation, such as appointment systems, deputising services, single-handed practitioners or primary care emergency centres, are related to the demand for out-of-hours care or the increasing demands on A&E departments.[15]

As well as variation within local areas, it is also likely that the number of calls varies around the country. General practices operate very differently in different areas and patients have differing characteristics and expectations. It would be surprising if the level of demand for out-of-hours care were the same in inner London and in rural Wales. At present, little is known about this issue, but one should beware of generalising from the experience in one area when planning services in another.

A sophisticated understanding of the factors which underlie the varying demand for out-of-hours primary care is necessary in order to increase the appropriate use of services. This is important to individuals as well as to those funding healthcare. For health services, the medicalisation of out-of-hours calls for non-urgent symptoms leads to an increase in the use of healthcare facilities and an unjustifiable increase in expenditure. For the patient, this is also undesirable since it generates unnecessary anxiety and dependency.

The increase in demand

A number of research studies have calculated rates of night visits and out-of-hours calls in different years, settings and areas. Although this evidence should be interpreted cautiously for the reasons discussed above, the overall results suggest that there has been a long-term increase in demand for care over several decades. This increase will have had a marked effect on the working life of a general practitioner within the length of his or her career. A specific fee for carrying out a night visit was introduced in 1967. A typical doctor entering general practice in that year might have expected to make a night visit about once every six weeks. By the time, they retired 30 years later, they could expect to make a visit during the night about once a week. This may cause significant disruption not only to their sleep pattern but also to their ability to work effectively in the daytime.

This trend of increasing demand over time is not unique to the United Kingdom. Many countries have faced problems in designing a system of out-of-hours care to cope with rising demand. An ideal system would be accessible, provide high-quality care for urgent problems, support rather than detract from daytime services, be affordable and be acceptable to both patients and doctors. Achieving these aims in the face of limited resources and increasing expectations is a challenge in the context of out-of-hours care as it is for many other aspects of health service planning.

In some ways, all countries face the same dilemmas, but in other ways each country is unique. The principles of understanding the balance between supply and demand in terms of characteristics of the local population and of the supply of services apply in all settings. However, the models which are proposed to solve the problems are clearly related to the rest of the health-care system. Although the attempts made elsewhere to resolve the problems are interesting, comparisons between the UK and other countries are of limited value because of the different traditions in daytime primary care. This is particularly true in terms of the provision of out-of-hours care. In most countries (with notable exceptions such as The Netherlands) there is less emphasis on continuity of care from one general practice, home visits in the daytime are rare and telephone advice is common. A major challenge in each country is to design a system which integrates with the daytime primary care service. The above differences highlight the fact that different solutions may be appropriate in the context of the overall healthcare system.

The changing expectations of patients and doctors

The level of demand on the health service is related to patients' expectations, as well as to their level of illness and to the socioeconomic factors listed previously. These expectations are largely conditioned by previous experiences, which are in turn related to the supply of services. Therefore, the level of health service activity cannot be considered a measure of the need for services, as activity is a function of this balance between supply and demand. There have been a number of important social and political trends affecting both patients' and doctors' expectations which may have influenced the demand on out-of-hours services.

Changing patient expectations

The 1990 GP Contract and the 1989 NHS White Paper reflected a philosophy of consumerism, which encouraged patients to have increasingly high expectations of the health service. This was in keeping with a much wider change in society from which the health service was not exempt. Many service industries had responded to consumer demand over the previous decade by increasing opening hours and accessibility. Convenience stores opened from early morning to late at night, shops opened on Sundays and 24-hour telephone banking and all-hours petrol stations became commonplace. It would be surprising if this had no effect on the demand for primary healthcare.

Over the period between 1966 and 1990, many aspects of general practice organisation developed and it is possible that some of these changes could have had an impact on patients' demands for out-of-hours care. The increasing use of appointment systems may have led to reduced availability of GPs in the daytime and this may have precipitated an increasing number of calls after doctors' surgeries were closed. It has also been suggested that the use of deputising services led to an increase in out-of-hours calls, as patients learnt that they could expect a home visit virtually on request. Conversely, if patients prefer to contact a doctor they know, the use of an unknown deputy could have prevented some calls if patients decided to wait until their surgery reopened. As previously described, the evidence for an inflationary effect from the use of deputising services is inconsistent.

Change in the attitudes of doctors and in the medical workforce

The increasing demand from patients was met by an increasing reluctance from general practitioners to work at night, leading to serious dissatisfaction within the medical profession and demands for change. The most important stimulus to change in the attitudes and expectations of doctors was probably the 1990 GP Contract, which not only had a direct effect on night visiting but also had an impact on many other aspects of primary care, the role of GPs and, more subtly, on their attitude to their work. The financial disincentives against using deputising services created by this new Contract provoked an angry response from doctors, particularly in deprived areas, who had come to rely on those services. This led doctors to question whether it was really necessary or advantageous for patients to be visited at night by a doctor who knew them. Heath[18] suggested that the philosophy of the market engendered by the Contract led GPs to consider the financial value attributed to various aspects of their work and this resulted in an 'attrition of vocation'.

> 'As patients became consumers, doctors became purveyors of a commodity rather than members of a vocational profession providing a public service. They then begin to look at precisely what they are paid for offering a 24 hour service 365 days of the year and they find that it is very little for the discomfort of having to get out of a warm bed after a long day's work and with the prospect of another one only a few hours away.'

The extent to which GPs resented out-of-hours work became clear when the GMSC undertook a major national survey of all GPs in the UK in 1992.[19] Almost 25 000 doctors replied, a response rate of 70%. More than half the respondents disagreed that 24-hour responsibility should remain an integral feature of general practice, 82% thought it should be possible to opt out and 73% of doctors personally wished to opt out. The opposition to the 24-hour commitment was most marked amongst younger GPs.

The strength of feeling which was apparent from this survey gave support to those who argued for a political campaign to change GPs' terms of service, a campaign which led to threats of mass resignation and eventually to some contractual changes. Why had GPs become so unwilling to continue their 24-hour responsibility for patient care?

First, there had been a long-term trend for GPs to decrease their personal commitment to out-of-hours work in terms of the number of hours spent on call.[20] The demand from doctors for shorter working hours and greater leisure time reflects the same trend in other areas of society.

Second, doctors who qualified before the mid-1980s had been trained into a profession which accepted long hours on call as the norm, having worked every other night or every third night as a hospital doctor. During the 1980s, the issue of junior hospital doctors' working hours became highly politicised. Doctors who entered general practice regarded frequent on-call duties as exploitative, rather than an essential feature of medicine, and were unwilling to accept partnerships in practices which involved onerous rota commitments. Amid growing recruitment difficulties, out-of-hours work was perceived to be one of the most important negative aspects deterring doctors from entering general practice.[21]

Third, there were important changes in the medical workforce. Between 1983 and 1995 the proportion of women doctors increased from 17% to 30% and 31% of these principals were part time.[22] Many of these doctors had domestic commitments and were seeking to work more defined hours.

Fourth, women doctors particularly, but also their male colleagues, increasingly expressed concern about the rise of aggression and actual violence when working at night. A survey in 1991 found that most general practitioners had experienced abuse or violence in the previous 12 months. There had been 90 incidents of assault and 37 physical injuries, of which 22 (66%) occurred during night calls.[23] One response to the fear of violence was to increase the use of deputising services.

The changes in the medical workforce, in the nature of general practice and in the 1990 GP Contract may have led to subtle changes in how GPs viewed their professional responsibilities. It is clear from articles written in the 1970s and 1980s that the delivery of out-of-hours care within a small practice rota was assumed to represent good practice, as it embodied the concept of personal and continuing care which was central to the professional values of general practice. The use of deputising services was at best a necessary evil. In many regions of the country, practices which used deputising services were not considered suitable to undertake vocational training of GPs. However, by the 1990s, general practitioners were redefining the nature of professional responsibility and suggesting that personal 24-hour care was unnecessary, inefficient and possibly harmful. Iliffe and Haug[24] argued that the demand for 24-hour care was unrealistic and fuelled ideas of omnipotence in doctors. They asserted that it was impossible to justify disturbing the sleep of GPs, thus making them tired the next day and effectively wasting a precious and expensive resource, for the sake of one or two calls.[24]

The attempts by GPs to change their contractual arrangements and devise new models of out-of-hours care can be seen as a creative response to the challenges of meeting the demands of patients. A negative manifestation of their unwillingness or inability to meet these demands was the evidence of poor morale in general practice and difficulties in recruiting young doctors. The reluctance of general practitioners to offer out-of-hours care may have been partly due to their general demoralisation after the imposition of the 1990 Contract. The 24-hour commitment was only one further stress for doctors who were facing many new demands, for example in health promotion and in purchasing secondary care.

Increasing concern about out-of-hours care led to the threat of industrial action by GPs. Negotiations eventually resulted in several changes, including a restructuring of the payment system for night visits. This removed the differential fees which penalised doctors who delegated visits to deputising services or co-operatives. Other changes included a patient education campaign to encourage appropriate use of the out-of-hours service, an agreement to identify a national price for the out-of-hours component of GP workload and a new right for GPs to transfer their out-of-hours responsibilities to another GP principal. The government also instituted a £45 million development fund to support new initiatives such as primary care centres.

The incentives created by these changes seemed likely to lead to a growth in centralised out-of-hours care provided by co-operatives and deputising services, with fewer GPs making visits personally. Earlier changes to the GP's terms of service had made the doctor responsible for deciding whether and where a consultation should take place, which was likely to lead to more telephone advice and primary care centre consultations and fewer home visits. By 1995, therefore, the combination of financial support and more flexible regulations had created the conditions necessary for a period of innovation in developing new ways of delivering 24-hour primary care. These innovations came about in response to pressure from doctors for change in the system because of a perception of increasing demand, the changing expectations of both patients and doctors and changes in the medical workforce.

References

1   Salisbury C (1993) Visiting through the night. *BMJ.* **306**: 762–4.

2   Brogan C, Eveling D, Fairman S, Gray A, Pickard D (1996) *Evaluation of Out of Hours Services.* Buckinghamshire Health Board, Aylesbury.

3   Kai J (1996) What worries parents when their preschool children are acutely ill, and why: a qualitative study. *BMJ.* **313**: 983–6.

4   Hopton J, Hogg R, McKee I (1996) Patients' accounts of calling the doctor out of hours: qualitative study in one general practice. *BMJ.* **313**: 991–4.

5   Singh S (1988) Self-referral to accident and emergency department: patients' perceptions. *BMJ.* **297**: 1179–80.

6   Brogan C, Pickard D, Gray A, Fairman S, Hill A (1998) The use of out of hours services: a cross sectional survey. *BMJ.* **316**: 524–7.

7   Carlisle R, Groom LM, Avery AJ, Boot D, Earwicker S (1998) Relation of out of hours activity by general practice and accident and emergency services with deprivation in Nottingham: longitudinal survey. *BMJ.* **316**: 520–3.

8   Shipman C, Longhurst S, Hollenbach F, Dale J (1997) Using out-of-hours services: general practice or A&E? *Family Pract.* **14**: 503–9.

9   Majeed FA, Cook DG, Hilton S, Poloniecki J, Hagen A (1995) Annual night visiting rates in 129 general practices in one family health services authority: association with patient and general practice characteristics. *Br J Gen Pract.* **45**: 531–5.

10   Lang T, Davido A, Diakité B *et al.* (1996) Non-urgent care in the hospital medical emergency department in France: how much and which health needs does it reflect? *J Epidemiol Commun Health.* **50**: 456–62.

11   Selby JV, Fireman BH, Swain BE (1996) Effect of a co-payment on use of the emergency department in a health maintenance organisation. *NEJM.* **334**: 635–41.

12   O'Grady KF, Manning WG, Newhouse JP, Brook RH (1985) The impact of cost sharing on emergency department use. *NEJM.* **313**: 484–90.

13   Boerma WGW, Fleming DM (1998) *The Role of General Practice in Systems of Health Care.* WHO/Stationery Office, London.

14   Olesen F, Jolleys JV (1994) Out of hours service: the Danish solution examined. *BMJ.* **309**: 1624–6.

15   Roberts E, Mays N (1997) *Accident and Emergency Care at the Primary–Secondary Care Interface: a systematic review of the evidence on substitution.* King's Fund, London.

16   Whynes D, Baines D (1996) Explaining variations in the frequency of night visits in general practice. *Family Pract.* **13**: 174–8.

17   Usherwood TP, Kapasi MA, Barber JH (1985) Wide variations in the night visiting rate. *J R Coll Gen Pract.* **35**: 395.

18   Heath I (1995) *The Mystery of General Practice.* Nuffield Provincial Hospitals Trust, London.

19   Electoral Reform Ballot Services (1992) *Your Choices for the Future: a survey of GP opinion, UK report.* ERBS, London.

20   Hallam, L. (1994) Primary medical care outside normal working hours: review of published work. *BMJ.* **308**: 249–53.

21   Rowsell R, Morgan M, Sarangi J (1995) General practitioner registrars' views about a career in general practice. *Br J Gen Pract.* **45**: 601–4.

22   Anonymous (1995) *General Medical Services Statistics for England and Wales.* HMSO, London.

23   Hobbs FD (1991) Violence in general practice: a survey of general practitioners' views. *BMJ.* **302**: 329–32.

24   Iliffe S, Haug U (1991) Out of hours work in general practice. *BMJ.* **302**: 1584–6.

CHAPTER THREE

A framework of models of out-of-hours general practice care

Chris Salisbury

In order to consider the most appropriate way to provide out-of-hours general practice care, it is helpful to disentangle the characteristics of the *providers* of care from the different *means* (forms of care or settings) in which care is delivered. For example, it is possible to compare the advantages and disadvantages of home visits and telephone advice, as different means of providing out-of-hours care. It is also possible to compare the relative merits of alternative providers, such as deputising services or GP co-operatives.

Different providers may offer a different range of services; for example, some may be more or less likely to offer telephone advice. Conversely, different providers may appear to offer the same type of care, but this may not have the same effects. Telephone advice offered by a GP who knows a patient well may be very different from telephone advice offered by a nurse working to a protocol at a central advice centre.

This chapter sets out a framework for considering out-of-hours care based on the different settings for care and the different types of organisation which provide care.

Settings for care

Home visits

Until recently, most patients contacting a GP outside surgery hours would have expected to receive a visit to their home. The home visit therefore came to be seen as the standard against which other forms of care should be judged. The conservative view (reflected in the advice of the medical defence societies) until recently was that general practitioners could not fulfil their responsibilities to their patients unless they conducted a face-to-face consultation with any patient who requested one. Most doctors provided out-of-hours care within a local practice rota and once surgeries were closed, this usually meant that patients received home visits.

In routine daytime general practice there has been a gradual decline in the number of home visits over many years. Almost a quarter (22%) of consultations in 1971 occurred in patients' homes; by 1990 this figure had reduced to 10%.[1] This trend has been mirrored in out-of-hours care by an increasing interest in alternatives to home visits, such as telephone advice and attendance at primary care centres.

There are several claimed advantages to home visits. If it is assumed that most out-of-hours calls are for patients who believe themselves to be very unwell, then patients can be assessed without being moved. It is also possible to assess people in their own environment, which may help doctors to understand the psychosocial context of an illness. Some patients request home visits because they have no transport to take them to a primary care centre.

However, home visits are extremely costly in terms of a doctor's time, taking about three times as long as a typical surgery consultation. They are expensive not only in terms of professional time, but also in travel costs. Home visits have other disadvantages as a setting for conducting consultations. It is difficult to examine a patient in a poorly lit bedroom, often with distractions due to televisions, barking dogs and noise from children. Doctors are also reluctant to visit patients at home because of the fear of violence and a concern that they are particularly vulnerable targets because they are assumed to be carrying drugs.

Many doctors would argue that patients who claim to need home visits because they are too ill to travel find it quite possible to attend A&E departments and that seriously ill patients are likely to have to travel to hospital for admission in any event. The issue of appropriate grounds for home visits has been contentious and highlights the fact that decisions about appropriate out-of-hours care depend not only on evidence of effectiveness, but also on consideration of the balance between the priorities of patients and professionals.

It may be that there are certain groups of patients for whom home visits are justifiable and the most appropriate form of care. The National Association of GP Co-operatives has offered guidance about when to offer home visits (Box 3.1), with a view to increased consistency in decisions, which in turn will ultimately influence patients' expectations. These expectations may change over time, but the appropriate use of visits is likely to continue to be a focus for debate.

Box 3.1: NAGPC Visiting Guidelines

National Association of GP Co-operatives
Central Office
511 Etruria Road, Basford
Stoke on Trent
Staffordshire, ST4 6HT

Tel: 0113 275 8361 Fax: 0113 275 8676

NAGPC Information Sheet

Visiting Guidelines

'**Medical Emergency**' in general practice constitutes a condition which in the reasonable medical opinion would result in undue distress, harm or considerable suffering if not seen before surgery opening hours.

The NAGPC council has considered these guidelines, produced by the North Staffs co-op, local GPs and their LMC. We believe they are eminently sensible and we are grateful to be given the chance to adopt them. You may wish to copy them to your GP members, or simply put them on your notice board.

Basic Principles

1 Terms of Service: The modification to the GP's contractual arrangement came into force in February 1995. Paragraph 13 of these amended regulations clearly states that in the case of a patient whose 'condition is such', it is for the doctor to decide, based on 'the doctor's reasonable opinion', as to whether the patient should attend a doctor's premises or be visited at home.

It is also very important to emphasise that it is specifically stated in paragraph 13, that there is nothing in the Terms of Service that prevents a doctor referring a patient directly to hospital without first seeing them, providing 'the medical condition of the patient makes that course of action appropriate'.

2 General practice has never been, and can never be, an emergency service along the lines of police or ambulance services. There is neither the manpower, infrastructure nor communications to work in this way. To try and work this way would inevitably harm other aspects of our work. We cannot provide an emergency response service when we are scrubbed up providing minor surgery to our patients. Neither is it appropriate for a doctor to feel compelled to leave a busy pre-booked surgery to attend a patient at home, whom it would seem may be suffering from a serious medical emergency. It is likely that the doctor will contribute little to the patient's care above and beyond that offered by the paramedics. Waiting for him/her to attend may well cause ultimate delay in hospital treatment and, in addition, major disruptions to the surgery timetable.

Box 3.1: Continued

3 In the guidelines, no distinction between 'in hours' and 'out of hours' has been made. The 'rules' governing where treatment takes place apply equally well in and out of hours. Once again it is for a doctor to decide, based on 'reasonable opinion', as to whether a consultation needs to take place before the patient could be seen within normal hours (paragraph 13 of the Terms of Service).

4 Throughout the development of these guidelines, the quality of medical care offered by general practitioners to their patients has been of paramount importance. The emphasis is that clinical effectiveness must, in some circumstances, take precedence over patient convenience.

Clarification and examples of visiting guidelines in action
1 Situation where GP home visiting makes clinical sense and provides the best way to give a medical opinion:

- the terminally ill
- the truly bedbound patient to whom travel to premises by car would cause a deterioration in medical condition or unacceptable discomfort.

2 Situations where on occasions visiting may be useful.
Where, after initial assessment over the telephone, a seriously ill patient may be helped by a GP and other commitments do not prevent him/her from arriving prior to the ambulance. Examples of such situations are:

- myocardial infarction
- severe shortness of breath
- severe haemorrhage.

It must be understood that if a GP is about to embark on a booked surgery of 25 patients and is informed that one of his/her patients is suffering from symptoms suggestive of a myocardial infarct, the sensible approach may well be to arrange paramedical ambulance rather than attend personally.

3 Situations where visiting is not usually required:

- common symptoms of childhood, fevers, cold, cough, earache, headache, diarrhoea/vomiting and most cases of abdominal pain. These patients are almost always well enough to travel by car. The old wives' tale that it is unwise to take a child out with a fever is blatantly untrue. It may well be that these children are not indeed fit to travel by bus or walk, but car transport is sensible and always available from friends, relatives or taxi firms
- adults with common problems of cough, sore throat and 'flu-like' symptoms.

Reproduced with permission from the National Association of GP Co-operatives.

Primary care centres

Primary care centres (PCCs) are centralised consulting facilities, open in the evenings and weekends or throughout the night. The establishment of primary care centres has been one of the most important developments in recent years. Primary care centres may be simply an arrangement to open one local surgery outside normal hours, staffed by general practitioners working in an extended rota. Alternatively, they may be fully equipped consulting suites (possibly purpose built), often in general hospitals close to A&E departments, staffed by several doctors, nurses and receptionists.

A large proportion of out-of-hours calls concern young children and common presenting complaints include upper respiratory tract infections, ear infections and gastrointestinal conditions. Such patients can readily be transported to primary care centres. General practitioners are strongly supportive of this idea, which increases their efficiency and offers them better facilities for interviewing and examining patients. It may also be that doctors feel more comfortable in an environment which feels familiar.

GP co-operatives have particularly pioneered the development of primary care centres, but many commercial deputising services have followed suit. In 1995 the government introduced several measures to support the shift towards premises-based out-of-hours care. These include changes in the GPs' terms of service, alterations to the night visit fee structure and a development fund to support the establishment of new primary care centres.

Initial evaluations suggested that the success of these centres was limited, with many patients declining to attend because of a lack of transport or because they felt too ill.[2] Although doctors were enthusiastic about centre-based care, patients appeared to be more ambivalent. The proportion of patients agreeing to attend primary care centres is very variable and the reasons for this are unclear. Relevant factors may include the position and accessibility of the centre, the proximity of alternative sources of help such as A&E departments, the quality of the facilities and the policies of the receptionists and doctors with regard to inviting patients to attend.

There is considerable debate whether or not primary care centres should be situated next to hospital A&E departments. The advantages are that hospitals are usually well known and accessible and that it may be possible to encourage patients to attend the most appropriate venue. Patients presenting with primary care problems in A&E can be redirected to the PCC and trauma patients can be transferred in the opposite direction. Disadvantages include the potential for a transfer of workload without a corresponding transfer of resources. There may also be problems in terms of managing demand. Most primary care centres only accept patients who have been invited to attend following a telephone assessment, whereas A&E departments permit open access. In addition, receptionists at some co-operatives invite any caller who is willing and able to attend the primary care centre to do so, with a view to reducing the demands on the doctors or nurses offering telephone advice. Providing consultations in this way, conveniently avoiding the need for patients to make an appointment during the day, seems likely to accelerate demand for out-of-hours primary care.

The issue of providing transport services to enable patients to attend primary care centres is also contentious. Lack of transport is the most common reason that patients give for declining to attend a primary care centre. The argument for providing transport services is that this reduces the need for home visits. By contrast, it can be argued that transport is usually available from local taxi companies if not from neighbours and friends. Although it may be claimed that this is too expensive, it is no less expensive to transport a doctor to the patient. The difference is that the cost is less visible. The relevant issue is not how patient transport should be arranged, but whether patients, doctors or the health service should be responsible for the costs.

Telephone advice

Increasing attention has been paid to the use of the telephone for advice and assessment. General practitioners have provided telephone advice to out-of-hours callers for many years, but the increasing importance of this form of care raises several issues, some of which are briefly discussed here. Telephone triage provided by nurses is described more fully in Chapter Seven.

The first issue concerns the purpose of the consultation. Some patients telephone during the out-of-hours period to obtain advice. They are not seeking a face-to-face consultation, but may need reassurance or guidance about self-management. This type of consultation is distinct from telephone triage, as a means of managing demand. This implies that the doctor or nurse is assessing whether or not they feel the caller needs a consultation at a centre or their home or can be managed with telephone advice alone. Patients may not necessarily receive the type of care they were requesting.

The second question concerns the safety of telephone triage, particularly if patients expressly request a home visit. It is clearly important to demonstrate that it is possible to make a telephone assessment of a patient's problem without a serious risk of an adverse outcome. Towards this end, many organisations have introduced computerised protocols for the management of common illnesses. The use of such protocols helps to ensure a consistent level of quality of advice and provides a structured record to demonstrate that a full assessment has been made.

A third question is whether it matters if doctors or nurses offer telephone consultations, in terms of safety, cost-effectiveness and acceptability to patients.

What is the appropriate level of training needed to offer telephone advice? Protocols as described above were particularly developed to help nurses involved in the telephone triage of out-of-hours callers. In the USA the concept of nurses advising telephone callers has been developed with considerable sophistication. Access Health, based in California, is a 24-hour telephone 'personal health management service'. People subscribe to managed care plans of various types, paid by monthly instalments, and at a time of need the subscriber has one 24-hour telephone access point to all healthcare information and services. On contacting the service, a nurse can help the patient decide the best way of obtaining help with their problem which will be covered by their particular level of care plan. Nurses have access to computerised databases of health information, drug formularies and clinical guidelines. Using protocols, they advise many patients themselves. The nurses can also connect callers to pre-recorded advice tapes on a number of health topics. The service aims only to help subscribers obtain appropriate help but it also constrains costs by restricting use of the hospital emergency room, which has been the traditional provider of out-of-hours care in the USA. Similar ideas for a single telephone number through which callers can gain access to appropriate out-of-hours care has led to the introduction of NHS Direct, as discussed below.

A fourth issue concerns the acceptability of telephone advice to patients. Although telephone consultations are popular with doctors because they reduce the number of home visits and are very time efficient, there is some evidence that patients have reservations. Experience both in the UK and in Denmark suggests that patients are less satisfied with telephone consultations than with home visits or attendance at a primary care centre.[3,4] This is particularly the case if they had expected to receive a home visit. The system of out-of-hours care in Denmark was reformed in 1992, leading to a service which provided incentives for doctors to provide telephone advice and discouraged home visits. There was an initial decline in patient satisfaction, but this later improved as patients became accustomed to the new system.

The fifth consideration is the effect on overall demand of an easily accessible out-of-hours telephone advice service. Although doctors have been concerned about the rising demand for care, the number of calls outside surgery hours is still very small as a proportion of the total primary care workload. Many patients are very reluctant to 'bother' a doctor outside normal hours. The promotion of a free professional advice service, easily available 24 hours a day, is likely to lead to a further rise in demand. It is difficult to predict the size of this increase, but the total number of calls could multiply several fold.

The framework of providers

The above section has outlined some of the issues pertaining to home visits, primary care centres and telephone advice. The following section outlines a framework of providers of care. This provides a brief overview of the claimed advantages and disadvantages of each model of organisation, as a background to Part Two of this book.

Personal or practice rota care

Before the growth of commercial deputising services in the 1960s, the GP's 24-hour responsibility meant providing care personally or in a practice rota. Since many more practitioners were single-handed or in small practices, this entailed frequent nights on call. This meant that a large proportion of out-of-hours consultations involved doctors and patients who knew each other. It was argued that this continuity of care was one of the cardinal features of general practice. The advantages of continuity of care include the fact that the doctor may have personal knowledge of the patient, their relevant medical history and their social situation. Even if the doctor does not know the patient personally, he or she has easy access to their notes and can discuss them with other colleagues in the primary healthcare team. This enhanced integration with the daytime primary care service and made it possible to offer consistent policies of care. These arguments led many to believe that providing out-of-hours care within a practice rota (rather than using a deputising service) was one of the markers of high-quality general practice. But to what extent are these arguments valid?

As practices became larger and larger, it was increasingly common for a visiting doctor to have no previous knowledge of the patient. Although in theory the GP could have access to the medical records, few doctors would make an extra journey during the night to collect the notes. The issues of communication, quality and consistency of care can all be overcome with appropriate organisation. Although patients appear to prefer to see a doctor from their own practice rather than a deputy, this may be partly related to expectation.

The arguments about the value of personal care are part of a wider debate about the core values of general practice. Although many doctors remained ambivalent and gained satisfaction from providing a traditional personal service, the rise in patient demand, the pressures for change described in Chapters One and Two and the growth of GP co-operatives have combined to cause a rapid decline in the number of GPs providing practice rota care.

Deputising services

A deputising service can be defined as a commercial organisation which provides out-of-hours care on behalf of subscribing GPs. Deputising services were originally established in the late 1950s and expanded rapidly in the 1960s and 1970s to cover most large towns, so that by 1984 45% of all GPs nationally subscribed to them.[5] The increasing contribution of deputising services caused controversy amongst both professionals and public. The arguments against these services included claims that they led to an increase in night visits, that they employed overworked and inappropriately trained deputies who provided inadequate care and that they undermined continuity of care. Each of these claims has been vigorously disputed. It is likely that deputising services enabled general practice to survive in areas where it would have been very difficult to recruit doctors to provide personal care on their own at night. Proponents of deputising services have argued that they provide an efficient system of call management, with the advantages of a large-scale organisation, and that their quality of care is monitored more closely than is the case with daytime general practice.

Deputising services have been subject to more intense scrutiny than other out-of-hours services, probably because of the controversy surrounding their use. The evidence about the various claims and counterclaims is discussed in Chapter Four.

GP co-operatives

A 'GP co-operative' has been defined as a 'non-profit making organisation entirely owned, and medically staffed by, the general practitioners of the area in which they operate'.[6] Co-operatives vary considerably in their size and level of organisation. Most provide telephone advice as well as home visits and many also provide an out-of-hours primary care centre to which patients can be invited.

The principal motivation behind the development of co-operatives was to enable GPs to be on call less often at night and for them to work more efficiently. Hobday had shown in 1984 that the night workload in one health district of almost 200 000 patients was only sufficient to justify involving two doctors, yet an average of 26 GPs were on call each night.[7] Working frequent nights on call interrupted by telephone calls causes a disproportionate level of disruption to the GP's life and his or her enthusiasm for work the following day. It is claimed that the out-of-hours care provided by co-operatives is similar to that provided by a practice rota since all those involved are GP principals.[6] Unlike deputising services, the doctors give telephone advice and visit only when medically necessary without a financial motive.

There are several other claims about the advantages of GP co-operatives over commercial deputising services. Responsibility for 24-hour care remains within the profession, which enables integration with daytime services and avoids duplication or gaps in services. It is claimed that GPs feel involved and committed to the service. Many apparently enjoy working for the co-operative as they experience a different kind of working environment with a high proportion of acutely ill patients. The involvement of GPs in their own organisation constrains costs. Those seeing patients feel accountable to their local colleagues, which may enhance quality of care. A further effect of the co-operative is that local GPs meet each other and work together on a joint project, which reduces isolation. If doctors delegate out-of-hours care to a deputy who is not a GP principal in the same area, they remain legally responsible, but doctors working in a co-operative are responsible for their own acts and omissions.

Co-operatives developed partly because of dissatisfaction with the cost and quality of care provided by deputising services and many of the doctors joining co-operatives would not have previously subscribed to a deputising service. However, it is arguable that the larger co-operatives need formalised organisational arrangements which make them very much like deputising services. It is debatable whether the care provided, as measured by process measures, quality of care and patient satisfaction, is more similar to a deputising service than a practice rota. The main criticism of deputising services has been the loss of continuity of care. It is interesting that co-operatives have not faced the same criticism. The growth of co-operatives has been supported by government and by local health authorities as well as by general practitioners. The reasons for this, and a more detailed description of this form of organisation, can be found in Chapter Five.

NHS Direct

In 1997, the Chief Medical Officer published a review of emergency services in the community.[8] One recommendation in his final report was the introduction and evaluation of a telephone helpline giving a single point of access to all out-of-hours health and social services. This recommendation has been implemented in the form of NHS Direct and pilot projects have been established in various centres around the country. Important questions which should be addressed by the evaluation include whether the greater accessibility offered by NHS Direct will further boost demand, the extent to which the service acts as triage rather than simply offering advice and particularly how NHS Direct will integrate with other providers of out-of-hours services. These issues are discussed in Part Three of this book.

References

1   OPCS (1992) *General Household Survey, 1990.* OPCS Social Survey Division, London.

2   Cragg DK, Campbell SM, Roland MO (1994) Out of hours primary care centres: characteristics of those attending and declining to attend. *BMJ.* **309**: 1627–9.

3   Salisbury C (1997) Postal survey of patients' satisfaction with a general practice out of hours cooperative. *BMJ.* **314**: 1594–8.

4   Christensen MB, Olesen F (1998) Out of hours service in Denmark: evaluation five years after reform. *BMJ.* **316**: 1502–5.

5   Anonymous (1984) Deputising services: a serious blunder [editorial]. *BMJ.* **288**: 172.

6   Reynolds M (1995) *Guidance from the National Association of GP Co-operatives.* NAGPC, Aylesford, Kent.

7   Hobday PJ (1984) Night workload in one health district. *BMJ.* **289**: 663–4.

8   Calman K (1997) *Developing Emergency Services in the Community. The Final Report.* NHS Executive, London.

PART TWO

Models of organisation

Introduction

In Part One, we set the scene and developed an agenda of basic issues which confront funders, providers and users of primary care services outside normal surgery hours. We have explored the role of different professional groups in providing services and the ways in which they are managed and funded in a variety of European countries. We have highlighted the increasing tensions between the aspirations of patients and constraints on human and financial resources. We have also discussed at some length the issues of demand and supply and the increasingly divergent attitudes of patients and providers which are at the heart of this problem. In Chapter Three, we concentrated on general practitioner services in the UK within a framework based on the different settings in which care is provided and the different organisational models available.

In Part Two there are six chapters, five of which provide a detailed description and in-depth analysis of a particular form of service delivery. We look at the development, regulation and activities of commercial deputising services and at the ways in which they are responding to changes in legislation and the growth of GP co-operatives. A lengthy chapter is devoted to describing the various models of co-operative organisation, management, infrastructure, working patterns and funding arrangements. Patients' views of co-operative services are also examined. The role of the GP in A&E departments, the potential for developing this joint approach to care and the barriers which must be overcome before it is more widely adopted are explored in Chapter Seven. The increasing role being played by nurses is examined from two perspectives in Chapters Eight and Nine: the part they play in telephone triage and advice, and their central position in minor injury units.

Part Two concludes with a review of the care provided for specific groups of patients with particular needs, concentrating on palliative care for people who are chronically or terminally ill, patients with mental health problems, the homeless and those from different cultural backgrounds. Gaps in service provision are identified and suggestions for improvements made, with examples of existing efforts to answer the needs of these special groups.

Each chapter within the section provides evidence from evaluations, examples of good practice and suggestions as to where particular models of care might lead.

CHAPTER FOUR

Deputising services

Robert McKinley and David Cragg

A deputising service is a commercial organisation which contracts to provide out-of-hours care on behalf of general practitioners. The care is delivered by doctors employed by the service who are qualified and accredited for or have exceptional experience of primary care. The contract can specify the provision of some or all of this care. Traditionally, care was delivered at home but, more recently, deputising services have been offering telephone advice and centre-based consultations.

Development of deputising services

A major feature of general practice over the last 40 years has been the birth and subsequent growth of commercial deputising services. This is exemplified by the growth of the largest provider, Healthcall (Box 4.1). This commercial expansion is reflected in the actual usage of deputising services. In 1964, only 9% of general practitioners were reported to 'sometimes' use deputising

---

Box 4.1: Milestones in the development of Healthcall plc

1955 First service established in South London
1964 Services established in Manchester, Birmingham, Liverpool and Leeds
1966 Air-Call / BMA agreement with establishment of BMA duty doctor service in Sheffield
1976 BMA duty doctor services in 19 cities in England, Scotland and Wales
1984 Air-Call medical services de-merged from Air-Call
1990 Management buyout of Healthcall
1994 Flotation of Healthcall on the stock market, market valuation £56 million

services.[1] The number of GP subscribers to such services doubled between 1971 and 1976[2] and by 1977, 42% of general practitioners used a deputising service for 'at least some' of their out-of-hours work.[1] By 1993, there were deputising services operating in 81 of the 93 family health service authorities (FHSAs) in the United Kingdom and, in urban areas, 75% of general practitioners had been given permission to use them for at least part of their out-of-hours care. At that time deputising services performed one-third of all night visits nationally and two-thirds of night visits in inner-city areas, responding to over 1 million requests for care each year. By 1996, deputising services were operating in 100 cities in England, Scotland and Wales and held contracts with an estimated 14 000 general practitioners nationwide.[3] Nevertheless, the recent rapid expansion in the general practice out-of-hours co-operative movement means the expansion of commercial deputising services has probably peaked and further expansion is likely to be in the range of services provided.

Regulatory framework for deputising services

Guidelines were introduced in 1984 to regulate deputising services; these aimed to ensure that 'out-of-hours care in general practice, however it is provided, should be of no lesser standard than that provided in hours'. The guideline established a requirement for each FHSA (now health authority) to establish a deputising services subcommittee and to appoint a deputising service liaison officer. The deputising services subcommittee advised the FHSA on requests by general practitioners to use deputising services and to establish a code of practice for any services operating in its area. It was stated that the code of practice should include requirements for the deputising service to ensure the 'competence and sufficiency' of the doctors it employs, the provision of transport and communications facilities and how requests for care should be prioritised and the response to them. Adherence to the guidelines was nevertheless variable nationally.[4] In 1993, some FHSAs only required that they were notified by general practitioners of their intention to use a service while others had developed detailed service specifications which were effectively monitored.

Partly in response to the rapid growth of the co-operative movement, in 1997 the terms of service for general practitioners were amended. Subscribing general practitioners were required to take all reasonable steps to ensure that the service provided by any organisation which provided deputies would be adequate and appropriate, paying particular regard to the interests of their patients. The omission of a definition for a deputising service meant that all such organisations were included. Thus, almost all the responsibility for monitoring their actions was transferred to the subscribing general practitioner.

The requirement to notify the health authority of the intention to delegate care remained but not consent to do so. Health authorities retained the power to terminate such delegation of care.

General description of the activities of a deputising service

Deputising services provide a mix of services. The 'switchboard' often acts as an 'answering service' for subscribers as well as receiving requests for out-of-hours care and passing them to the appropriate deputy who provides direct care to patients. Traditionally, the response to almost all requests for care was to provide a domiciliary visit, a practice which has been much criticised. More recently, deputising services have been expanding their repertoire of responses to requests for care and now also provide telephone advice, either from doctors or nurses, or out-of-hours centres which patients may attend for care. This pattern of provision is evolving rapidly and there are few national data to indicate the proportions of each type of care provided.

The nature of the contract between the subscribing general practitioner and the deputising service varies. It may provide for the payment of a fee for each request for care dealt with by the deputising service on an occasional basis or the payment of an annuity for the handling of all requests for out-of-hours care. Therefore, the extent of the delegation of care by the practitioner could vary from parts of occasional nights through the year to delegating all requests for out-of-hours care after the health centre closes on weekdays until the following morning and throughout the weekend.

Although deputising services are paid directly by subscribing general practitioners for providing out-of-hours services, general practitioners currently receive an annual allowance for the provision of out-of-hours care and an item-of-service fee which is paid for each face-to-face consultation carried out by or on behalf of the general practitioner between 10.00 pm and 8.00 am. Thus general practitioners can offset at least part of the expense of delegating their care to a deputising service.

Evaluation of deputising services

Although deputising services had become a major provider of out-of-hours care and the dominant commercial force in the market by the early 1990s, this did not occur without opposition to and criticism of their work. In 1976 the Royal College of General Practitioners believed that the organisation of doctors into local rotas was likely to be 'preferable to delegation as a method of providing out-of-hours care and relieving doctors of their commitment to provide care 24 hours a day'.[5] Others have adopted strong stances, believing that general practitioners who use deputising services are 'doing a disservice to their patients and to general practice as a whole'.[6] It was postulated that although deputising services could provide a competent clinical service, they could not match the care given to patients by practice doctors in terms of their 'experience, commitment and local knowledge' and therefore the care they provided was 'second best'. Nevertheless, the wider body of professional concern was more moderate. In 1984, 86% of respondents to a questionnaire were opposed to restriction of the usage of deputising services by general practitioners but gave overall support for a minimum requirement for experience for deputies.[7]

> *A senior partner from this practice recently told me that a commercial deputising service now handles all (night) calls. His views have changed: he believes that being on call is unprofessional. It betokens a serious failure to maintain personal and professional boundaries and encourages doctors to develop self-destructive fantasies of omnipotence and omniavailability.[8]*

There is now a significant body of research on the activities of deputising services which allows us to appraise several aspects of their work. Some of the most important studies, on which this chapter is based, are summarised in Table 4.1. To set these data in context, we have compared them to data from a number of evaluations of out-of-hours care provided by practices. Practice-based care is at one end of a continuum from 'absolute' continuity of medical out-of-hours care to total delegation which is exemplified by deputising services. Data from evaluations of other models of out-of-hours care are presented in Chapters Five to Eight.

Process of care

Types of care provided

Historically, descriptive studies have reported that the vast majority of care provided by deputising services was as a home visit; indeed, all but one study showed that fewer than 10% of patients received telephone advice. Practice doctors providing their own out-of-hours care give more telephone advice but there is considerable variation between reports in the proportion of telephone advice provided (18–49%). The only randomised controlled trial comparing deputising services with own-practice doctors providing out-of-hours care

Table 4.1: Summary of research on care provided by deputising services and practice doctors and the outcomes on which this chapter is based

	Authors	Title	Reference	Study group Deputising services (D), Practices (P), Single/Multiple (S/M)	Methods Descriptive (D) Comparative (C) RCT (R)	Results used Response (R)* Delay (D) Prescribing (P)	Hospital referral (H) Satisfaction (S) Outcome (O)
1	Bain DJG	Deputising services: the Portsmouth experience.	BMJ 1984;**289**: 471–473	D,S	D	R,D,P,H	
2	Bollam MJ, McCarthy M, Modell M	Patients' assessment of out of hours care in general practice.	BMJ 1988;**296**: 829–832	DPM	D	D,P,S	
3	Cartwright A, Anderson A	General practice revisited.	London: Tavistock, 1981			S	
4	Cragg DK, Campbell SM, Roland MO.	Out of hours primary care centres: characteristics of those attending and declining to attend.	BMJ 1994;**309**: 1627–1629	D,M	R	R,D,M,H,S Attendance rate	
5	Cragg DK, McKinley RK, Roland MO. et al.	Comparison of out of hours care provided by patients' own general practitioners and commercial deputising services: a randomised controlled trial. I: The process of care.	BMJ 1997;**314**: 187–189	D,P,M	R	R,D,P,H	
6	Crowe MGF, Hurwood DS, Taylor RW	Out-of-hours calls in a Leicestershire practice.	BMJ 1976;**1**: 1582–1584	P,S	D	R,P,H	

Table 4.1: Continued

Authors	Title	Reference	Study group Deputising services (D). Practices (P), Single/Multiple (S/M)	Methods Descriptive (D) Comparative (C) RCT (R)	Results used Response (R)* Delay (D) Prescribing (P)	Hospital referral (H) Satisfaction (S) Outcome (O)
7 Dixon RA, Williams BT	Twelve months of deputising: 100,000 patient contacts with eighteen services.	BMJ 1977;**1**: 560–563	D,M	D	R,D,P,H Change in request rate	
8 Dixon RA, Williams BT	Patient satisfaction with general practitioner deputising services.	BMJ 1988;**297**: 1519–1522	DM	D	D,H,S Patient expectation	
9 Gadsby R	Telephone advice in managing out-of-hours care.	J R Coll Gen Pract 1987;**37**:462	P,S	D	R	
10 Lockstone DR	Night calls in a group practice.	J R Coll Gen Pract 1976;**26**:68–71	D,S	D	R	
11 Marsh GN, Horne RA, Channing DM	A study of telephone advice in managing out-of-hours calls.	J R Coll Gen Pract 1987;**37**:301–304	P,S	D	R,H,O	
12 McCarthy M, Bollam MJ	Telephone advice of out of hours calls in general practice.	Br J Gen Pract 1990; **40**:19–21	D,P,M	D	R,H Use of deputising	
13 McKinley RK, Cragg DK, Hastings AM, et al.	Comparison of out of hours care provided by patients' own general practitioners and commercial deputising services: a randomised controlled trial. II: The outcome of care.	BMJ 1997;**314**: 190–193	D,P,M	R	S,O	

Table 4.1: Continued

Authors	Title	Reference	Study group Deputising services (D), Practices (P), Single/Multiple (S/M)	Methods Descriptive (D) Comparative (C) RCT (R)	Results used Response (R)* Delay (D) Prescribing (P)	Hospital referral (H) Satisfaction (S) Outcome (O)
14 Morrison WG, Pennycook AG	A study of the content of general practitioners' referral letters to an accident and emergency department.	Br J Clin Pract 1991;**45**:95–96	D,P,M	C	H	
15 Murray TS, Barber JH	The workload of a commercial deputising service.	J R Coll Gen Pract 1977;**27**:209–211	D,S	D	H	
16 Pitts J, Whitby M	Out of hours workload of a suburban general practice: deprivation or expectation?	BMJ 1990;**300**:1113–1115	D,S	D	R,H	
17 Prudhoe RH	Deputising services.	BMJ 1984;**288**:718	P,S	C	S	
18 Riddell JA	Out of hours visits in a group practice.	BMJ 1980;1518–1519	P,S	D	H	
19 Ridsdill Smith RM	Out-of-hours calls.	Update 1983;274–277	P,S	D	R,P,H	
20 Rutherford WH, Bell JSE	Comparison of the patient populations referred to the accident and emergency department outside working hours by general practitioners and by their deputising services.	Resuscitation 1975;**4**:271–278	Patients referred to an A&E department	Comparison of referrals from practice and deputising doctors	R	

Table 4.1: Continued

Authors	Title	Reference	Study group Deputising services (D), Practices (P), Single/Multiple (S/M)	Methods Descriptive (D) Comparative (C) RCT (R)	Results used Response (R)* Delay (D) Prescribing (P) Hospital referral (H) Satisfaction (S) Outcome (O)
21 Sawyer L, Arber S	Changes in home visiting and night and weekend cover: the patient's view.	*BMJ* 1982:**284**: 1531–1534			D,S
22 Stevenson JSK	Advantages of deputising services: a personal view.	*BMJ* 1982:**284**: 947–949	P,S	D	R,D,H,O
23 Tulloch AJ	Out-of-hours calls in an Oxfordshire practice.	*Practitioner* 1984; **228**:663–666	P,S	D	R
24 Whitby M, Freeman G	GPs' differing responses to out-of-hours calls.	*Practitioner* 1989; **233**:493–495	P,S	C	R,P,H
25 Williams BT, Dixon RA, Knowelden J	BMA deputising service in Sheffield.	*BMJ* 1973; **1**:593–599	D,S	D	R,D,P,R,H

Telephone advice, home visit or attendance at surgery/out-of-hours centre demonstrated that practice doctors were much more likely to give telephone advice than deputising doctors (22% vs 1% of calls).

Since the change in the regulations concerning payments for out-of-hours services, deputising services have started to provide more care at out-of-hours centres and more telephone advice. Nevertheless, as mentioned previously, few national data exist about the current proportions of each type of care provided although attendance rates in the 'five centres' study (number 5 in Table 4.1) varied from 9% to 52%. It is not known how representative these data are or how they compare with the results of practice-based care. (See studies numbered 1, 4–7, 9, 10–12, 16, 19, 20, 22–25 and 28 in Table 4.1.)

Delay between the request for care and the visit

In surveys of the work of deputising services, the delay between the request for care and the visit has often been described as the proportions of patients seen within one hour and within two hours. These appear to have remained relatively constant over the last 20 years. In 1973, the proportions were reported as 72% and 96% and in 1977 as 55% and 80%. In two studies in the 1980s, 67% and 60% were seen within one hour and 93% and 92% within two hours respectively. However, in one study in 1994 the proportions were 46% and 82% which may reflect the increasing difficulty services have in coping with demand.

Comparative studies demonstrate that practice doctors visit more quickly. For example, in a descriptive study in 1982, 87% of patients were seen by a practice doctor within one hour and 59% by deputies within one hour. The randomised controlled trial of deputising services versus practice doctors showed a median delay of 35 minutes between the request and visit for practice doctors and 52 minutes for deputising doctors. (See studies numbered 1, 2, 4, 5, 7, 8, 21, 22 and 25 in Table 4.1.)

Prescribing

Doctors who work for deputising services are perceived to 'overprescribe'. Descriptive studies suggest that deputising doctors prescribe to between 65 and 70% of patients who request care and practice doctors to between 30 and 35% of patients. Although the randomised controlled trial of deputising doctors versus practice doctors found practice doctors were less likely to prescribe than deputising doctors, the differences were smaller (56% vs 63%). Not only do practice doctors prescribe less, their prescriptions may be more appropriate. The randomised controlled trial showed that they were less likely to prescribe antibiotics (44% vs 61% of prescriptions), more likely to prescribe generically (58% vs 31%) and a greater proportion of their prescriptions were from a pre-defined formulary of essential drugs for out-of-hours care (50% vs 41%). (See studies numbered 1, 2, 5–7, 19, 24 and 25 in Table 4.1.)

Hospital referral

The number of patients 'referred for admission' after a request for out-of-hours care has remained remarkably consistent over time between practice and deputising doctors. The proportion of patients referred for admission has remained at between 7% and 9% in multiple studies since 1973, except for one which reported an admission rate of 11%. Referral rates to A&E have been less frequently reported but have also remained between 4% and 5%. Descriptions of out-of-hours work carried out by own practice doctors reported between 5% and 10% of patients being referred to hospital for admission. The randomised controlled trial found no difference in the proportion of patients admitted to hospital or referred to A&E departments by deputising and practice doctors.

Similarly, indicators of the quality of hospital referrals show few differences in the performance of deputising and practice doctors. Studies of referral letters to A&E departments demonstrated that deputising doctors may actually provide more information in the letters than practice doctors. No differences have been demonstrated in the proportion of patients admitted after referral or the subsequent duration of the admission. (See studies numbered 1, 4–8, 11, 12, 14–16, 18, 20, 22, 24 and 25 in Table 4.1.)

Outcome of out-of-hours care

Patient satisfaction

An understanding of patient satisfaction with out-of-hours care is limited, first, by the use of poorly characterised satisfaction instruments and, second, by the lack of comparative data. Nevertheless, in descriptive studies of deputising services, large majorities of patients expressed overall satisfaction and satisfaction with specific aspects of the service. However, some comparative studies have suggested that patients were more satisfied with the care provided by practice doctors, a finding confirmed by the randomised controlled trial even when other differences between the services were controlled for. A consistent finding has been that patient satisfaction declines with increasing delay between the request for and provision of care. Satisfaction is also strongly related to age, with older people being more satisfied with care than younger people and the parents of young children.

It is less certain what determines the diminished satisfaction with the care provided by deputising doctors. The greater delay between the request for and provision of care may be relevant. Diminished satisfaction has also been attributed to perceptions that the deputising doctor was careless or tired, was unknown to the patient, had a poor command of English or that the consultation was rushed. (See studies numbered 2–4, 8, 13, 17 and 21 in Table 4.1.)

Health outcomes

Again, despite anecdotal concerns that deputising services provide inferior care, there are few data to substantiate this. In one report from a single practice, the care of 76% of patients who were seen by a deputising service in a year was reviewed; 70% required no further care related to the presenting episode while only one patient was dissatisfied with the care provided. The only randomised controlled trial of deputising services versus own-practice doctors showed no differences in the change in symptoms or overall health status measured between 24 and 120 hours after the request for care or in the subsequent use of the health services over the following two weeks. (See studies numbered 11, 13 and 21 in Table 4.1.)

Continuity of care

A major criticism of delegation of out-of-hours care has been that continuity of care between the patient and his or her usual doctor is disrupted. Nevertheless, there was no difference in expressed satisfaction with continuity of care in the randomised controlled trial. We have attributed this to a combination of low continuity of care between routine and out-of-hours care within practices providing their own care on a rota system and patients' perceptions of need for urgent medical care over-riding any desire for continuity of care. (See study number 13 in Table 4.1.)

Summary

The outcome of comparisons of out-of-hours care provided by deputising services and by patients' own practices is summarised in Box 4.2. The importance attached to these differences will vary according to the perceptions of the observer. Patients and their advocacy groups may consider delay and satisfaction most important while practices unable to meet the demand from their own patients for out-of-hours care and considering delegation may concentrate on the similarity of outcome of care. Nevertheless, it is important that any practice or provider which is considering delegating out-of-hours

---

Box 4.2:   Summary of comparisons between out-of-hours care provided by deputising and practice doctors

No difference in:
   health outcomes
   admission rates

Own-practice doctors:
   visit more quickly
   prescribe less
   patients are more satisfied
No systematically collected national data on the proportions of care provided as telephone advice, centre attendance or a home visit.

---

care is aware of the implications of their decisions for both patients and practice staff. It is also important that the community groups are aware of the relative benefits of care provided by patients' own general practitioners and the cost to those practitioners and practices of continuing to provide such a service.

Future development of deputising services

We anticipate changes in three main areas: first, the contribution of deputising to the 'basket' of provision of out-of-hours services; second, the relationships between deputising services and other providers of out-of-hours services; and lastly, issues surrounding quality.

Contribution to overall provision of out-of-hours care by deputising services

Until the early 1990s, the provision of out-of-hours primary medical care could have been characterised as domiciliary visits by deputising services or a combination of telephone advice and domiciliary visits provided by practitioners. The increasing reluctance of general practitioners to provide their own out-of-hours care, the difficulties experienced by deputising services in recruiting staff to provide out-of-hours care and the General Medical

Services Committee survey of general practitioners highlighted the need for change in this pattern of provision.[9] Over 80% of practitioners agreed that it should be possible to opt out of their out-of-hours responsibilities and 73% expressed a desire to do so. In 1992, the then Minister for Health suggested a network of primary care centres to which patients would be expected to travel for care rather than receiving home visits from a doctor. At the same time, the widely held perceptions of general practitioners that the almost inevitable home visit which followed a request for care to a deputising visit promoted patients' expectation of such care prompted general practitioners to encourage deputising services to offer more telephone advice. Many deputising services are now 'triaging' requests for care to telephone advice, centre attendance and domiciliary visits. Some are experimenting with advice and care provided by suitably trained nurses, others have experimented with the local GP providing advice but delegating callers requiring a face-to-face consultation to the deputising service. Similarly, some general practice out-of-hours cooperatives have subcontracted aspects of their care (particularly home visits) to the local deputising service. Thus, although the provision of care has become more complex, it may become more flexible and adaptable to the needs of particular communities and areas.

The launch of the NHS Direct telephone advice service provides an opportunity for deputising services to contract for this work. As the largest providers of out-of-hours care in the United Kingdom, they have unrivalled experience in this area and must be regarded as potential providers of this service

Relationship between providers of out-of-hours care

Although much of the growth of general practice co-operatives has been in areas which were not served by deputising services, invariably co-operatives will have eroded the subscriber base of some deputising services. Although this represents a commercial threat to the deputising service, relationships between co-operatives and deputising services operating on the same 'turf' can be co-operative; for example, as in Manchester where co-operatives are buying domiciliary care from the local deputising services. Nevertheless, this is not always the case. There have been anecdotal reports of some deputising services countering the perceived threat of the establishment of co-operatives in their areas by various means. These could take the form of undercutting the proposed subscriptions to co-operatives, thus undermining their financial base, or a declaration that the deputising service would no longer be viable if a co-operative was established. This could undermine local practitioners' confidence in the proposed co-operative by removing the possibility of them having a 'fallback' if it should fail.

Quality of care provided

With the institution of practice-based complaints mechanisms, patients who are dissatisfied with the care they receive from deputising services may complain to their own practice. With the development of clinical governance and the delegation of many of the responsibilities of health authorities to primary care groups, it is likely that the investigation of such complaints will exert a powerful force for change. We anticipate that such quality improvement initiatives will initially address delay and triage decisions if only because of their immediate importance to patients and the increasing voice patients will have within the health service. We also expect that prescribing and ensuring the continuing professional development of deputising service staff will be major 'professional' priorities.

Delay

The only routinely monitored quality indicator applied to out-of-hours care provided by deputising services has been the delay between the request for care and provision of care. This has the merits of simplicity of collection and importance to patients (as evidenced by the decline in satisfaction with increasing delay). Its major deficit is that achievement of a standard for the proportion of consultations completed within one hour of the request for care does not ensure that those who require urgent attention for medical emergencies do not experience inappropriate delay.

Prescribing

Increased attention is being paid to prescribing by deputising doctors. Some deputising services are now preparing out-of-hours formularies in an attempt to rationalise prescribing. Nevertheless, monitoring prescribing activity by deputising services will require significant extra activity by the services and it is uncertain whether this will be feasible.

Triage decisions

Most deputising services can report the proportion of requests for care which result in telephone advice, centre attendance or a home visit. Unfortunately, as with the delay until a visit, such data do not indicate whether or not triage to each type of care was appropriate. A major challenge for quality assurance for all providers of out-of-hours services will be to ensure that the cost implications of providing each type of care (telephone advice, centre attendance and home visits) do not inappropriately affect the choice of type of care offered to patients. Triage decisions will always require judgement by nurses or doctors. Although monitoring the appropriateness of such judgements will be difficult to institute, it is imperative to do so to ensure that the services retain the confidence of patients.

Continuing professional development and training for staff employed by deputising services

The change from near universal provision of domiciliary visits to active triage and allocation of patients to types of care which may not be immediately acceptable or desired creates new challenges for all deputising service staff. Services will have to ensure that, as a minimum, all telephonists and triage staff (whether nursing or medical) have good communication and negotiation skills in dealing with anxious people who may become angry if they are offered care which they perceive to be inappropriate.

Summary

Our view of the important issues which will face deputising services is summarised in Box 4.3. The formation of primary care groups and their adoption of responsibility for clinical governance will play a powerful role in shaping the future of out-of-hours services. Deputising services will have to respond to this new agenda. There is likely to be greater variability in arrangements between localities and deputising services will need to respond flexibly. Deputising services, along with all other providers, will need to demonstrate that they have well-trained staff who provide high-quality services to patients in their locality.

Box 4.3:   Summary: Deputising services, the future

- Changing relationships with other providers of out-of-hours services
- Flexible contribution to out-of-hours services
- Quality: appropriateness of
    triage
    delay
    prescribing
- Staff development and training

References

1   Cartwright A, Anderson A (1981) *General Practice Revisited.* Tavistock, London.

2   Gravelle HSE (1980) Deputising services, prescribing in general practice and dispensing in the community. King's Fund Centre, London.

3   Hallam L, Cragg D (1994) Organisation of primary care services outside normal working hours. *BMJ.* **309**: 1621–3.

4   Cragg D, Hallam L (1994) Quality standards for deputising services. *BMJ.* **309**: 1630.

5   Anonymous (1976) Out of hours work. *J R Coll Gen Pract.* **26**: 3–6.

6   Creighton P (1982) A case against deputising services. *BMJ.* **284**: 1089–91.

7   Wakeford R (1984) Deputies: who needs them? *World Med.* **223**: 493–5.

8   Hurwitz B (1994) Out of hours. *BMJ.* **309**: 1593–4.

9   General Medical Services Committee (1992) *Your Choices: Special Report.* GMSC, London.

CHAPTER FIVE

GP out-of-hours co-operatives

Lesley Hallam and Mark Reynolds

Introduction

The advent of co-operatives has transformed on-call provision and appears to have boosted the morale of GPs across much of the UK. In 1988 there were approximately 500 GPs in co-operatives. By 1998 there were 22 000. This chapter reviews the development of co-operatives in the context of the cultural, political and regulatory frameworks which influenced and affected their development and will continue to do so. Examples and descriptions of various models are given, together with some instances of good practice. The NHS is moving fast and co-operatives face changes with the advent of primary care groups (PCGs) and NHS Direct. The last section of this chapter therefore considers where this model is leading with these and other developments in view.

Definition

'A GP co-operative is a non-profit making organisation, entirely and equally owned by, and mostly medically staffed by the GP principals of the area in which it operates. The main purpose of such a co-op is to cover the "out-of-hours" commitments of its members.' (National Association of GP Co-operatives)

Most co-operatives are constituted and incorporated as companies limited by guarantee, without share capital and with individual liability among members set at a nominal sum. If income exceeds operating costs, the cash surplus is either returned to members, often in the form of shift payments, or used for further development. Each GP member has an equal vote in the organisation's affairs, with key decisions taken at general meetings.

The original belief that only GP principals should provide rota cover has been tempered in recent years, particularly in the light of training needs, and it is now unusual for registrars to be excluded. Rotas may also include longterm locums and recently qualified VTS doctors. Approximately 10% of co-operatives now have arrangements with commercial providers who cover some of their work. More rarely, directly employed doctors fill the most unpopular shifts.

As well as covering the out-of-hours commitments of members, co-operatives frequently organise educational and social activities for members. Some offer their telephone answering services to other professional groups as a means of raising income.

The influence of the regulatory framework

The key elements of the regulatory framework which have influenced co-operative development are as follows.

The *Red Book*

Rules which govern the reimbursement to GPs of the costs of ancillary staff, computing equipment and premises are contained in the *Red Book*. Family health service authorities (FHSAs) were responsible for their interpretation and application. Most FHSAs did not support the view that co-operatives were eligible for these General Medical Services (GMS) fund payments. Threatened legal action by the Association of Commercial Deputising Companies against FHSAs who held opposing views reinforced this negative interpretation of the rules. Co-operatives were thus dependent on members' contributions to meet the full costs of staff and infrastructure. Only recently and only in some areas have GMS funds become more widely available.

The higher rate night visit fee

In order to discourage the use of commercial deputising services, the government introduced a differential fee for night visits in 1990. GPs providing rota cover in groups of ten or less received £45 per visit; GPs using larger rotas or commercial services received only £15. Members of co-operatives thus suffered a fall in income. Existing co-operatives suffered and planned co-operatives failed to materialise until this situation was rectified in 1995 with the removal of the differential fee.

Paragraph 13, terms of service

Paragraph 13 of the GPs' terms of service relates to where services to patients should be rendered by GPs. In 1995 this paragraph was restated to clarify the GP's right to decide if, when and where an out-of-hours consultation should take place, on clinical grounds. Prior to this many GPs believed that refusal to visit a patient at home, no matter how trivial the problem, could leave them open to censure. Clarification facilitated the increased use of co-operative primary care centres. The issue of social need for a home visit (for instance, where patients lack transport) was and still is fudged, leading to uneasy compromises. Nonetheless, centre-based consultations are rising.

The development of co-operatives

The first co-operatives were set up in the late 1970s but there were only a handful prior to 1990, when social, cultural and health service changes produced a climate which favoured their development.

Demand for out-of-hours care rose steadily throughout the period. Studies suggest that in most areas it at least doubled and in some areas it tripled.[1] The percentage of serious medical conditions within the total number of calls decreased and GPs became increasingly irritated by the number of calls they perceived to be 'trivial'. Whilst GPs working in heavily urbanised areas were able to employ commercial deputising services to relieve them of the increasing burden of out-of-hours care, around 60% of GPs had no access to such services. They did their own on call, single-handed, within practices or in small rotas with neighbouring groups of GPs.[2,3]

In 1990, the imposition of a new Contract reduced GPs' professional autonomy, increased their daytime workload and resulted in considerable disenchantment with both their conditions of work and remuneration. Much of their anger became focused specifically on their 24-hour responsibilities.[4]

At the same time, Kent GPs were beginning to take up the co-operative idea, with the active support, both financial and moral, of their FHSA. Kent FHSA chose to interpret *Red Book* regulations to support its newly forming co-operatives, providing GMS funds for staff and infrastructure and publicly defending their decision to do so. East Anglia followed suit. The hitherto small National Association of General Practitioner Co-operatives (NAGPC) boosted its membership numbers considerably and became a significant voice in pressing for reforms to the regulatory framework which inhibited the development of co-operatives. Data collected by the Kent co-operatives from their inception proved invaluable in the political process. The GPs' traditional voice, the General Medical Services Committee (GMSC) of the British Medical Association (BMA), was effectively silenced in the early stages of the debate. A contract between the BMA and a commercial deputising service prevented them from supporting or promoting any other form of out-of-hours provision.

Reform of the regulatory framework and the creation of a ring-fenced fund of £45 million to support out-of-hours developments were finally realised in 1995. The existing co-operatives had by then demonstrated that they could:

- provide a low-cost service
- provide good-quality care and high levels of patient satisfaction
- relieve stress and improve the quality of personal life for GP members
- effectively cover rural and semirural areas as well as urban settings
- reduce GPs' sense of professional isolation, particularly when on call
- improve morale within the profession.

The out-of-hours development fund

The out-of-hours development fund provided the final catalyst for the spread of co-operatives. This fund was and is intended to facilitate the development of systems of care above the level of the practice which maintain or improve the quality of services to patients whilst alleviating stress on GPs. In theory, health authorities take a strategic view on quality, recruitment and patient services and allocate money to individual GPs for them to spend on a service if it meets the relevant criteria. It was not intended to be split equally among GPs, but in fact a per-GP share amounting to around £1400 became the norm, with varying top-ups from GMS funds. The fund allows bids for staff, premises, IT and other equipment. It precludes reimbursement of doctor-to-doctor payments and transport costs. The per-GP split and strict application of restrictions on use have produced underspends in some areas.

General description of the model

There is considerable diversity in the structure of co-operatives, the way in which they are managed and the patterns of care which they provide. In their formative stages, each co-operative adopts features of existing organisations which answer its needs within available resources. Where needs or resources differ, new infrastructures and systems are developed. Their evolution continues over time, reflecting greater experience and changing circumstances.

Box 5.1 illustrates the myriad differences between co-operatives in their composition and organisation. Differences in the patterns of care they provide are examined under 'Evidence from evaluations'.

Box 5.1:   Variation between co-operatives

Size
From ten GP members to over 400, covering from 12 000 patients to over 1 million. Larger co-operatives may be split into different constituencies, with varying degrees of autonomy. An average-sized co-operative will have between 70 and 80 members covering around 130 000 patients.

Area covered
From sparsely populated rural areas, through small market towns, to major conurbations. Some cover whole counties. Around two-thirds cover a mixture of urban and rural districts.

Management structure
From loosely knit 'clubs' in which all members carry equal responsibility for policy and operations to limited companies in which medical directors, paid administrators and managers are responsible to a management board and individual members may have limited influence.

Personnel
Administration, management, telephone answering, reception, triage and driving are variously carried out by GP members, subcontractors and employed staff. Small co-operatives may have little or no staff; large co-operatives can have payrolls of over 50.

GP rotas
In the smallest co-operatives, members usually have equal and fixed commitments to a rota, rarely receiving payment for duty periods. With increasing size comes increasing flexibility. Members frequently set their own level of commitment and receive payments reflecting the number, length and timing of their shifts. An average-sized co-operative will have two GPs on 'active' duty with a third in reserve, except for the 'graveyard' shift between midnight and 7.00 a.m. when only one GP may be on 'active' duty. At busy times there will be more.

Premises
Co-operatives covering large areas often run more than one emergency centre and may have a separate operational base. Centres are most commonly located in community hospitals, acute trust premises (including A&E departments and day clinics), community trust clinics, purpose-designed private buildings and members' surgeries. Domestic facilities for on-duty GPs and staff are sometimes poor.

Box 5.1:   Continued

Transport
Whilst some co-operatives rely on members driving their own vehicles, many own or lease vehicles and employ drivers. In some cases they offer patients transport to the emergency centre. Contracts with local ambulance trusts for cars and drivers are common.

Communications and records
Whilst services can and do operate with a mobile telephone and notepad, most use sophisticated communication and record systems, including call recording, computerised record systems with purpose-designed software, in-car terminals and printers, even satellite-based global positioning systems to track vehicles.

Finances
Co-operatives are supported by the out-of-hours development fund and membership subscriptions. Some receive additional health authority allowances for premises and staff. Income from contracts for telephone answering, administrative services or primary medical care services, for instance to a local A&E department, is limited. Their main expenditure headings are staff, premises, equipment and shift payments. Net costs of membership range from nil to around £4000 per annum per member.

Size and area covered

Co-operatives range in size from ten GP members to over 400. Human geography is a key factor in determining their size, structure and the area covered. An emergency centre can only provide a rapid response within a limited geographical area. Where that area has a high population density and many GPs, a large, single-centre co-operative offers members low rota commitments and low membership costs. Co-operatives covering rural districts with low population density tend to be either small or organised into sectors, each sector having its own centre. In either case, rota commitments are more onerous and operating costs per member can be much higher, particularly where several centres are needed.

Around two-thirds of co-operatives cover mixed urban and rural areas. The most common pattern is for their centre(s) to be based in the local market town(s) and for cover to extend to surrounding rural areas.

Management structure

The status of co-operatives ranges from loosely knit 'clubs' to limited companies. At its most formal, a co-operative will have a management board with elected members, sometimes representing individual constituencies within the co-operative. One or more medical directors/managers take responsibility for clinical issues, but may not always have voting rights. Where operational managers and administrators are employed, they report to the management board. A number of subcommittees, with elected or co-opted members, may have responsibilities for individual aspects of the co-operative's operations and development. They too will report back to the management board. An annual general meeting will be open to all members and any major policy decisions will normally be ratified or rejected in that forum.

At its most 'elite', a co-operative may be a limited company with two or three founders as its only directors and no representation on the board for the ordinary membership. They, as sole shareholders, have voting rights on major decisions at AGMs but have limited influence on day-to-day affairs.

At its most democratic, a small co-operative may hold regular meetings involving a representative from each member practice, with consensus decision making and collective responsibility.

'There is a great deal of democracy ... on the Committee most practices are represented and if the practice isn't, then there's a representative looking after their interests ... There's no excuse to feel your views are not being represented ... you've only got to speak to your partner who sits on the Committee.' (Member, small-town co-operative)

Avenues by which 'ordinary' members can receive information and make their views known include working groups, questionnaires and surveys, open meetings, constituency meetings, newsletters and informal lines of communication. The extent to which 'ordinary' members of a co-operative are and wish to be involved varies, both between co-operatives and between individual members.

'It's just a matter of "as long as the driver turns up and I turn up"; that's all that matters to me.' (Member, mid-sized, multisector co-operative)

Personnel

It is becoming increasingly unusual for co-operatives to function without any employed or subcontracted support personnel. Larger co-operatives, particularly those which are able to operate from a single centre, can have an impressive range of staff supporting their activities. Typically, they will have administrative or management support. Administrators and managers may themselves be supported by secretaries and record clerks. Not all co-operatives are self-managed. The most common external providers of managerial support are other co-operatives, community health service trusts and ambulance trusts.

Emergency centre staff commonly include telephonists/receptionists and drivers. In around a quarter of co-operatives there is some nursing support, notably to provide telephone triage and advice services. Frequently, nurses are employed through a contract with an NHS provider rather than employed direct. With a small number of members or a large number of centres, it may not be economically viable to employ a full complement of centre staff. In such situations, GPs themselves undertake these tasks or they are subcontracted. Again, other co-operatives, ambulance trusts and commercial message-handling services are the most common subcontractors.

Although nearly 90% of co-operatives are medically staffed wholly by their own members, it has become increasingly common in large urban areas for co-operatives and commercial deputising services to operate jointly. For instance, all night-time home visits may be carried out by deputies or centres may be staffed by deputies at night. More rarely, co-operatives directly employ doctors who routinely cover a number of unpopular shifts.

GP rotas

Organising the rota is possibly the most contentious aspect of co-operative management from the members' viewpoint and certainly one of the most frustrating and difficult tasks for administrators and managers. An initial, broad distinction must be made between those co-operatives which make payments to members based on the actual number of shifts they undertake and those which do not. Shift payment systems offer members the opportunity to set a preferred balance between membership costs and time commitments. They can be complicated, with a range of different tariffs reflecting the length and relative unpopularity of certain shifts. Tariffs may escalate over time when organisers experience difficulties filling particular rota 'slots'.

> 'We don't want to coerce people into working ... and the way to make them feel they want to work is to increase the price. The payments sometimes have to be increased at difficult times, like Christmas. Some co-operatives insist that you work three or four times a month, but we let people decide; find their own level and let the commercial rewards sort it out.' (Director, mid-sized co-operative covering mixed area)

In co-operatives where there are no shift payments, shifts are commonly allocated to practices, who in turn allocate them to individual partners. Again, they are commonly graded to reflect their relative unpopularity, with each practice responsible for a certain number of each grade. The number of shifts to be worked may be calculated on list size, number of partners, actual out-of-hours workload generated or some combination of these. All co-operative members thus do their 'fair share' of duty periods. The system is simpler than shift payments in accounting terms, but more complex in terms of setting the rota and less flexible for members.

Co-operative size has a considerable impact on members' rota commitments. Since it is impossible to have less than one GP on duty, in small and multicentre co-operatives the number of members rather than the level of demand for care dictates commitments. For example, in one co-operative of 75 GPs covering 120 000 patients from a single centre, each member works an average of 1.5 shifts per month. In another rural co-operative of 25 GPs covering 45 000 patients and operating two centres, the average commitment is 5.2 shifts per month.

Premises

Few co-operatives are fortunate enough to begin with natural bases for their operations. The exceptions are likely to be those covering rural areas where the GPs have historically used community or cottage hospitals to see primary care patients out of hours. Co-operatives covering rural areas without community hospitals may have difficulty finding convenient, independent bases for their operations and so rely on sharing a member practice's surgery accommodation. This also applies to some urban co-operatives. Over 20% of co-operatives are based in daytime health centre and surgery premises.

Purpose-designed centres, either new-builds or conversions, are rarely an option within co-operatives' limited budgets and under 10% have such facilities. Instead, a variety of buildings serving other, health-related purposes are pressed into service. Predominantly, these include hospital buildings, particularly those housing facilities which only operate during weekdays (around 45% of co-operatives), and acute hospital A&E departments (around 15%). The remainder share accommodation with services ranging from occupational and community health clinics to fire stations.

It follows that most co-operatives have good facilities for receiving and treating patients, but some have limited office and domestic facilities for staff and on-duty GPs.

'We have a camp bed to sleep in. The room is always miles too hot, and there's a toilet that flushes every 20 minutes down the corridor. It's awful.'

'We need to have a proper bedroom and a light and telephone table and that sort of thing. We have a camp bed and sleeping bag ... there are various tricks, like unplugging the fridge, sticking a piece of wood in [the toilet flushing mechanism], but really ...' (Members of one sector of a large co-operative covering a mainly rural area)

Transport

The liveried vehicles of GP co-operatives are becoming an increasingly common sight on Britain's roads. They may be owned by the co-operative, leased or provided under contract by an ambulance trust, who will also supply drivers.

Cars are predominantly used to transport GPs to patients' homes when a home visit is deemed necessary. More rarely, they also transport patients to centres, but relatively few co-operatives offer this service on a regular basis.

The 1998 review of GP out-of-hours services in Scotland suggested the desirability of providing transport for patients in rural areas. This is in line with the policy of the National Association of GP Co-operatives, but such costs are not currently allowable in bids for development fund money.

Communications and records

Whilst it is possible for a small co-operative to operate with a single telephone line, a pager and pad-and-pencil records, systems are frequently much more complex, with back-up and fail-safe mechanisms in place.

Communications must be maintained between large numbers of patients and the operational base or centre. Where there is more than one centre, they may be linked electronically. Operational bases and centres are linked to mobile GPs through combinations of two-way radios, mobile telephones, pagers and in-car computer terminals. Many larger co-operatives even have satellite-based global positioning systems in their vehicles.

Patients' telephone calls may be voice-recorded, for medicolegal purposes. Purpose-designed computer software can ensure that all patient contacts are logged and dealt with promptly and appropriately. Postcoding systems check that addresses are recorded correctly. Faxes or computer terminals link centres with member practices, ensuring that information on patient contacts passes between them.

Smaller and multicentre co-operatives sometimes choose to contract out communications, often to the local ambulance service, rather than invest heavily in hardware, software, licences and lines. Alternatively, one large co-operative may act as an umbrella organisation for a number of smaller ones. Commercial deputising services also have the necessary infrastructure to handle communications and records, but these relationships seldom last due to the inherent competition between the two types of system.

Finances

There is extensive variation between co-operatives in their operating costs, not only overall, which might be expected in the light of differences in size, but also in terms of their costs per GP member and per 1000 patients covered. There are also wide variations in the actual cost of membership to individual GPs. Whilst co-operatives' policies on shift payments for on-duty GPs are a factor, substantial differences still remain when this has been taken into account. Excluding shift costs, costs per member as low as £1080 and as high as £3800 were recently reported.[5] With the exception of shift payments, the major items of recurrent expenditure can be divided into four broad headings: directly employed staff and professional fees; transportation; communications; centre and office accommodation.

Major sources of income include annual grants from the out-of-hours development fund and, for some co-operatives, rent allowances and partial reimbursement of staff costs from their health authority. A few generate substantial sums from providing message-handling, administrative or clinical services to other organisations.

Membership subscriptions make up any shortfall between income and expenditure. Many co-operatives choose to concentrate their resources within particular expenditure headings at the expense of others, in order to minimise the costs which members must bear. Some operate on a shoestring in order to match operational costs and development fund income.

Evidence from evaluations of co-operatives and the care they provide

Most studies of GP co-operatives have been purely descriptive. An annual survey provides an overview of their structure, policy, management and patterns of service delivery.[6] Papers describing the operations of a single co-operative occasionally appear in refereed journals.[7-9] There are also frequent references to their activities in the popular medical press. Evaluative studies are rare and not easily accessible. This chapter thus relies heavily on two evaluative studies[5,10] and the authors' extensive knowledge and experience of out-of-hours co-operatives.

Setting up

There are a number of 'enabling' factors which appear to ease the formation of co-operatives and contribute to their success in maintaining operations (Box 5.2).

Box 5.2:   Enabling factors

* Strong commitment and leadership from founding GPs
* A sense of ownership amongst members
* Pre-existing links between local practices
* Natural geographical boundaries within which to operate
* Role models in neighbouring or similar geographical areas
* Lack of competition for patients between practices
* Extra financial and logistical support from health authorities
* Lack of competing, commercial services

There are several examples of planned co-operatives failing to materialise through lack of a 'product champion', interpractice rivalries and tensions, inappropriately drawn boundaries and poor financial support or management. Where there are alternative services available, these become more attractive in the face of such problems.

Area covered

Co-operatives which cover mixed areas, with some urban and some rural practices, represent around two-thirds of those in existence. The great majority manage their affairs to the satisfaction of both groups. However, they face potential problems reconciling conflicting perceptions and priorities. Urban GPs may be unhappy about the distances they are required to cover answering rural patients' needs, whilst rural GPs fear their patients will be unfairly denied home visits. Rural GPs may have greater concerns about their own safety when visiting deprived urban areas, whilst urban GPs see dark country lanes as inherently more dangerous.

If it is necessary to provide additional rural centres, there will be fewer GPs attached to rural centres than to an urban centre. Their rota commitments will be greater though their membership costs may remain the same. Maintaining more than one centre can increase operating costs significantly and since rural centres are usually more expensive per capita, one group may feel it is subsidising another. Such tensions can lead to fragmentation and even disintegration.

'[Cost per call out] is about £5 a patient in [x sector] and it rises to £20 or £25 in [y sector]. Clearly that means that one group of doctors is subsidising another. As I am at the expensive end of the scale, I would say that was reasonable, because it isn't my fault that I've got patients in a rural area. But obviously, *the doctors at the other end will say why should they subsidise us and I think that is a difficult thing to resolve.'* (Member, large sectorised co-operative covering mixed area)

Management structures and rota arrangements may need to be devised which ensure equal representation and amicable rota divisions among urban and rural GPs.

Additional problems are likely to surface where commercial deputising services exist within the co-operative's boundaries. Competition for subscribers can be fierce. The loss of urban members to a deputising service may threaten the viability of the co-operative for rural members who have no access to a commercial service.

Membership

In areas where population density is high and there are many GPs, the participation of all local GPs is less vital than in areas where population density is low and there are few GPs.

'The most difficult thing, particularly within a small rural area, is [that] for the co-operative to be effective, you have to have most of the people [GPs] involved. Otherwise, it's not viable. It's not like starting up a co-operative in a city where if one in four agree, that's fine. The problem here is the geographical spread ... you have got to get everyone in. It's an advanced exercise in politics ... It took quite a number of meetings and quite a bit of time.' (Founding member, small rural co-operative covering large area)

Somewhat perversely, individual practices on the periphery of a small co-operative's boundaries may be deliberately excluded from membership. The added area they represent can increase the number of GPs needed on duty, may require a second centre and hence will increase the rota commitments of existing members.

Recruiting a viable number of GP members often requires considerable effort and diplomacy on the part of a few highly committed individuals. A variety of circumstances influence success or failure (Box 5.3).

Asking local GPs to commit themselves to the idea of a co-operative and to work together on its development risks fluctuating levels of commitment as evolving plans become more or less acceptable to some. However, placing a firm proposal or business plan on the table at an introductory meeting risks alienating some prospective members who dislike particular aspects of the plan.

Where GPs are relatively content with their current arrangements for providing out-of-hours cover (for instance, in a joint rota with neighbouring

---

Box 5.3:   Key issues in recruiting GP members

- Timing
- Existing out-of-hours arrangements
- Demonstration that the service will be safe and effective
- Projected costs of membership
- Projected level of rota commitment
- Admission of individual partners or whole practices only
- Practice commitment to continuity of care

---

practices or using a commercial deputising service), the co-operative must offer them additional attractions: for example, further reductions in rota commitments, a higher quality service or cost savings. The costs of membership must be sufficiently low or the current demands of providing cover sufficiently high to make co-operative membership an attractive proposition.

Whilst there may be some scope for accepting partial membership from practices, this has to be limited. Having many practices in which only one or two partners are co-operative members will produce large swings in the number of patients being covered which are difficult to manage. It is thus unusual for some partners to stay outside the co-operative whilst others join.

Emergency centres

The limited availability of premises suitable for co-operative operations, particularly in rural areas, has already been mentioned. So too has the often prohibitive cost of building or converting premises. As a result, many co-operatives operate under less than ideal conditions in locations they would not otherwise have chosen.

> '... we only use a clinic which is used by other people at other times; it's not solely ours, which is not surprising because we only use it for short periods, and they [the hospital] feel that the alterations we want will interfere with their day-to-day running.' (Member, small co-operative based in a fracture clinic)

Some of the most common problems of sharing space with daytime users are shown in Box 5.4, though not all will apply in all circumstances.

There are some shared arrangements which work well, especially when purpose built to house both services.

Around 60% of co-operatives use acute hospital trust premises. Where they are based in day units, they are likely to face some of the problems listed

> **Box 5.4:**   Problems of shared space
>
> - Disconnecting and reconnecting computing and communications equipment daily
> - Competing with extracurricular meetings of daytime users for common room space
> - Inappropriate night-time security systems
> - Inadequate office and domestic facilities
> - No sleeping accommodation
> - No daytime office accommodation for administrative and clerical staff
> - Overlaps with over-running daytime services

in Box 5.4. Where they are located within A&E or casualty departments, they may face overcrowding, limited space, confusion between patient streams and tensions between hospital and primary care staff. There are, however, some advantages (Box 5.5).

> **Box 5.5:**   Advantages of hospital sites
>
> - Well-signposted, central location
> - Adequate parking
> - Access to clinical equipment
> - Help from hospital staff
> - 24-hour security
> - Improved GP–hospital doctor relations

Set against these advantages, location on an acute hospital site, in or near an A&E department, carries the risk of 'overmedicalising' minor problems by asking patients to come to a hospital. It can also blur the boundary between A&E services and primary care services. A&E staff may fear both an increase and a reduction in their workload due to the proximity of a 'part-time' primary care centre, dependent upon whether they are fully stretched or need the primary care workload to retain their viability. GPs fear an increased workload due to cross referrals from A&E and the higher visibility of their centre.

Co-operatives which receive cost-rent allowances for premises from their health authority have fewer financial constraints influencing their choice of location.

Structure and management

Whilst there is no evidence to suggest that there is an optimal size of co-operative, there are a number of organisational factors which appear to give 'added value' to members (Box 5.6).

Box 5.6:   'Added value'

- Bringing together 20–25 practices in a single centre
- Involving members as much as possible in setting policy
- Informing members about day-to-day affairs
- Employing staff who form the 'backbone' of the organisation
- Providing regular opportunities for interaction between members
- Extending activities to include educational and social meetings

---

A sense of 'ownership' among members distinguishes a truly co-operative enterprise from one which is more akin to a non-commercial deputising service. Involving and informing members and creating opportunities for interaction foster this sense of ownership. It is more difficult to attain in co-operatives which operate in sectors from multiple small centres. Single-GP duty rosters provide little opportunity for daily interaction and links with the wider organisation can be tenuous. A single centre with two or three GPs on duty together, a stable core of support staff and readily accessible directors and managers will experience less difficulty.

Personnel

One of the arguments in favour of employing staff and providing key services in-house is that it strengthens the co-operative's identity and reduces the sense of isolation experienced by an on-duty GP. Unfortunately, it is precisely those co-operatives which have the greatest need for added continuity and reduced isolation which are least likely to be able to afford it. With limited funds and multiple centres, central message handling becomes an attractive alternative to employing telephone and reception staff at each centre.

A central message-handling service may delay contact between patient and GP and so may be less acceptable to patients. Message handlers may not be aware of what is happening at a distant centre and so may not be able to adjust their responses accordingly. In a commercial service, the co-operative is likely to be only one of a number of clients and may get a poorer service than they would like. Most co-operatives eventually take this task on themselves.

Though the majority of co-operatives have drivers, it is not accepted by all that drivers are essential to their operations. Often they are seen as something of a luxury. Some GPs argue that their own vehicles, driving and navigation skills are superior and that their co-operative could operate more cheaply without drivers. Nonetheless, numerous advantages have been cited for having drivers (Box 5.7).

Box 5.7:   Advantages of having drivers

- Relieve GPs from the strain of driving and navigating
- Familiar with the territory through experience
- Provide added security for GP, car and equipment
- Reduce the sense of isolation and stress for GP
- Have the ability to fill other roles
- Provide continuity at centres where no other staff are employed
- Take responsibility for maintaining vehicles
- Undertake message handling

Drivers are expensive and may be idle for much of the night at centres with a low volume of night visiting. Whilst their job descriptions can be broadened if they are co-operative employees, this is unlikely to be the case if drivers and vehicles are subcontracted from ambulance trusts.

The relative merits of subcontracting and direct employment include the following.

Subcontracting
- No recruitment/training to undertake
- No payroll functions to undertake
- No rotas to set
- No need to purchase/lease vehicles

Direct employment
- Control over recruitment and training
- Flexible roles and responsibilities
- Flexible hours and times of duty
- First loyalty to the co-operative

The comments of a subcontracted driver employed by an ambulance trust hint at the problems of subcontracting from a driver's viewpoint.

'It's like being a lighthouse keeper. I do my set of shifts and disappear, [another driver] does his and disappears. We see each other at weekends when we do a

cross-over. We leave each other notes. It's lonely because of the command system; we don't have anyone to go to if we've got a problem ... even though our relationship on a day-to-day basis with the doctors is good.' (Driver for a sectorised, rural co-operative with no other centre staff)

Employing nurses to triage patients' calls and give telephone advice where necessary can significantly reduce doctors' workload. In a recent evaluation of a trial of nurse triage, nurses handled nearly 40% of out-of-hours callers without referral to a general practitioner.[11] However, nurses are expensive and they will only reduce the rota commitments of GPs if there would otherwise be two or three doctors on call. When there would normally only be one, that doctor must still be at the centre, albeit handling fewer calls. A study published in the *BMJ* recently demonstrated that trained, experienced nurses dealt with 50% of incoming calls as safely and effectively as the member GPs.[12]

Finances

The striking differences between co-operatives in their operating costs per member have already been discussed. The role played in this by shift payments has also been pointed out.

There is considerable disagreement on whether GPs should be paid by the co-operative for rota duties. Some see shift payments as an unnecessary complication which increases administrative workload. They rely on all members making an equal contribution to operating costs and rota commitments. Others argue that co-operatives which make shift payments are more accurately reflecting the true cost of providing out-of-hours services rather than contributing to the notion that it is a low-cost option. To some extent, their motives are political. However, shift payments do give members flexibility in their commitments and reward those who take a larger share of the work.

Whether or not shift payments are made, the net cost of membership is an important consideration for individual GPs. High net costs can destabilise co-operatives. If net costs increase, members leave in order to save money, increasing the subscriptions and often the rota commitments of those who remain. In areas with some deputising service cover, the deputising service may become an attractive alternative, without the necessity of working shifts at all.

'.... to actually run it costs us personally vast sums of money. Last year it was £3700. That was a bad patch ... There's a chap just now had to pull out because he can't afford it. To actually be faced with paying to provide a service

to the public is a joke, really, a bad joke.' (Member, mid-sized, sectorised co-operative covering rural areas)

Levels of demand and patterns of service delivery

It is not possible to assess objectively the impact that co-operatives have had on overall levels of demand for out-of-hours care. Accurate workload data prior to the formation of a co-operative are not generally available. Further, most have experienced changes in membership over time so that any such data would no longer be a valid point of comparison. Rising demand is believed to be part of a national trend and the impact of co-operative, centre-based care cannot be separated from the broader picture. Views are mixed. Some GP members believe that their co-operative has reduced demand, primarily by reducing home visiting. Others believe it has had no impact, whilst a significant number believe that centre-based care is fuelling demand by giving out-of-hours care a higher profile and making it more accessible to patients.

It seems clear that telephone consultations are increasing, centre attendances are increasing and home visiting is decreasing over time. There are striking variations between co-operatives in the pattern of care that they provide. Telephone advice may be given to as few as 20% or as many as 60% of patients. Between 20% and 50% of patients are asked to attend a centre. As few as 10% of patients may be visited at home or as many as 50%. The average seems to be around 40% telephone advice, 30% centre consultations and 25% home visits, with the remainder receiving some other form of care (e.g. admission or A&E referral).

The patients' view

A recent postal survey of 2400 out-of-hours consulters from six co-operatives revealed that the most common expectation among patients remained that they would be visited at home (43% of those with clear expectations) and only 18% of patients expected to be asked to attend a centre. Of 1865 open-ended responses to the question 'How do you feel, in general, about patients being invited to come in and see a doctor outside surgery hours?', 1396 (75%) were negative. Broadly, there were three overarching reasons why they felt they should not be asked to attend:

- the belief that people who call the doctor out-of-hours are too ill to travel
- the fact that the patient and others around him/her should not be inconvenienced, particularly by the need to arrange transport and childcare

- the belief that patients should have the option of being visited at home if they wish.

Over a third of those asked to attend a centre either refused (11%) or agreed reluctantly (26%).

Nonetheless, satisfaction levels with centre attendance were high. On three aspects (reception, waiting time at the centre and treatment received), around two-thirds expressed themselves as 'very satisfied' and only 5–7% as 'not very' or 'not at all' satisfied. Satisfaction with waiting times was lower for those visited at home (52% 'very' satisfied; 10% 'not very' or 'not at all' satisfied), but satisfaction with treatment at home was similar to centre attendances (66% and 8%). It is difficult to compare these satisfaction levels with those found in earlier studies of non co-operative care. Surgery attendances are rarely mentioned, different scales are used and deputising services are frequently involved.[13-16] Deputising services have generally been less satisfactory to patients. For instance, Dixon and Williams[17] reported that between 12% and 19% of their patient sample were dissatisfied with some aspect of their consultation with a deputy and 21% were dissatisfied with the time they waited for the deputy to arrive.

Telephone advice appears to be the least popular form of care received from the co-operatives. Only 44% of patients receiving telephone advice were 'very happy' with the advice they received and 22% were 'not very' or 'not at all' happy. However, this contrasts with the experiences of long-established co-operatives in Kent, who report that only around 10% of patients say they are not satisfied when asked a simple yes/no question.

Impact on other providers

There is no hard evidence on the impact which co-operatives have had on other providers of emergency services. Anecdote and interview surveys suggest that demand for all emergency services has risen in recent years and that much of this is viewed as inappropriate or misdirected. However, it does not seem that any one service is worsening or improving matters for another. A number of ways in which co-operatives might lead to higher A&E and/or ambulance workloads have been suggested, including:

- increases in referrals for unknown patients or when services are under pressure
- decreases in minor trauma work among rural GP members
- patients' unwillingness to transport themselves to a primary care centre
- difficulties in accessing busy co-operatives by telephone
- patient dissatisfaction with telephone advice
- distances creating unacceptable delays in the GP reaching a patient.

Conversely, co-operatives might have the opposite effect, through:

- accepting 'primary care' referrals from A&E departments
- providing a more accessible, higher profile primary care service
- shorter waiting times at centres than for 'low priority' A&E attenders
- on-duty GPs less likely than on-call GPs to refer as a matter of convenience.

It is likely that any small effects would balance each other out.

There is nothing to suggest that co-operatives should have any effect on community nursing services (much of whose work is pre-planned rather than emergency response), community psychiatric services, social services, dentistry or pharmacy.

Quality standards

As a consequence of a circular issued in 1984, responsibility for monitoring the performance of commercial deputising companies fell to FHSAs.[18] In fact, the guidelines were selectively implemented, with some FHSAs doing very little and others setting comprehensive standards which they expected the companies to meet.[19] Some health authorities treated co-operatives as if they were commercial companies and tried to implement the guidelines rigorously, though they were largely inappropriate. The circular was eventually scrapped and individual GPs are now responsible for ensuring that their out-of-hours service has adequate administrative, communication and financial systems and that adequate standards of care are provided. This has been incorporated into Paragraph 22 of the GPs' terms of service.

Whilst most co-operatives provide members with data on response times and activity levels, the advent of systems of clinical governance may require more formal examination of the co-operative's activities. We suggest that the aspects of the service shown in Box 5.8 should be monitored.

Box 5.8:   Aspects of services to be monitored

- Adequacy of service with reference to the number of doctors on duty, the needs of the population and the nature of the area
- Transfer of clinical information to and from a patient's own doctor
- Training, performance and indemnification of employed supporting staff
- Transport arrangements
- Internal communication systems
- Communications with patients
- Assessment and prioritising of requests for care
- Criteria for giving telephone advice, centre-based consultations and home visits
- Record systems
- Complaints systems
- Remedial notices

A model of good practice

There are two main areas of activity within a co-operative: the clinical activity of the doctors and the activity of the supporting infrastructure. In terms of clinical activity, the variation amongst GPs is notable, particularly in thresholds for seeing patients. The service must cope with and respect these differences whilst trying to narrow the range of behaviours. GPs on duty will see and manage patients whom they may well never see again. Their lack of knowledge of outcomes and lack of feedback from patients and their families have important implications for training. Procedures that promote good clinical practice and guard against the results of failures need to be put in place.

The administrative structure should serve the clinical activity of the co-operative but, in addition, elements within the administrative structure can also promote a sense of ownership and camaraderie among members (Boxes 5.9 and 5.10).

Box 5.9: Examples of procedures that promote good clinical practice

Busy periods
Anticipate where possible and roster extra doctors; regularly update rotas in the light of changing demand patterns; always have a reserve doctor on call at home; overlap shifts to clear any call backlogs.

Outcome & feedback
Allow consulting doctor to select cases for feedback, contact patients' practices and provide brief notes of outcomes for consulting GP; provide individual GPs with comparative data on their triage decisions.

Satisfaction surveys
Randomly sample between 1-in-20 and 1-in-30 patients; send postal question-naire on access, response times, and doctor's performance; feed results back to the doctors concerned; identify areas where co-operative can improve.

Priority rating
Provide clear guidance to telephonists on 'rapid action' calls; monitor progress of urgent calls through the system; review performance and identify problems.

Communication with surgeries
Communicate important events by telephone as soon as surgeries open; use computerised, automated faxes where possible; keep surgery-provided management plans for 'special' patients.

Clinical protocols
Conformity is impossible, but consider frequent educational events as a more effective tool in reaching common standards.

Box 5.9:   Continued

Patients' notes
In complex cases, leave a summary with the patient.

Call recording
Record calls to establish facts in cases of complaint and to use as training tool.

Procedural protocols
Appoint shift leader to take decisions on calling in reserves; implement systems
for dealing with INT and TR claims; establish policies for drug abusers, drop-ins
and unusual events and document actions.

Interprofessional communication
Where possible, establish working relationships with other professional groups,
e.g. psychiatric rapid response teams, paramedics and district nursing services.

Box 5.10:   Examples of administrative structures that support clinical activity

Rota management
Incorporate flexibility to allow adaptation in busy times; always have reserves;
remind doctors of their duty sessions; introduce sanctions which encourage
punctuality.

Staff competence
Encourage multiskilling; provide training opportunities to improve quality and
morale.

Financial structure
Set basic subscription levels to provide an adequate income for the co-operative
independent of demand levels, e.g. by basing subscription levels on list sizes;
introduce a supplementary billing system for 'high demand' practices.

Computerisation
Have contingency plans to cover computer crashes and power failures.

Communications
Provide mobile, in-car, computer reception units to reduce delay, record arrival
times and provide speech-free car-to-base communication system; back these
up with mobile phones or radios.

Information and involvement
Seek members' views on their information needs; regularly disseminate co-
operative 'news'; promote a sense of ownership among members by involving
them in the co-operative's affairs.

Doctor behaviour
Leave as little administrative paperwork to the doctor as possible; ideally, doctors
should only have to fill in their clinical notes and the bare bones of response
times.

Important issues to consider in planning this type of service

Earlier sections in this chapter have highlighted a number of key issues which should be considered in planning this type of service. Briefly, these are as follows.

Is a co-operative viable in terms of numbers of prospective members and the geography of the area they serve?

• Areas with moderate or high population densities, many GPs and no alternatives to practice rota cover are most favourably placed.
• Covering an extensive area with a limited number of GPs will require added centres, increased rota commitments and higher membership costs but
• Rural areas are definitely feasible – witness Cornwall and Northumbria.
• There may be natural geographical boundaries which must be considered.

Is a co-operative viable in financial terms?

• Identify sources of funding and negotiate support from health authorities.
• Long-term financial planning is vital to the success of the operation.
• High membership costs can destabilise co-operatives.

Will the co-operative be able to meet demand for out-of-hours care effectively and efficiently?

• Assess existing demand for out-of-hours care.
• Estimate the number of GPs required on duty at the centre(s).

How will the co-operative create a sense of commitment and ownership?

• Set the level of membership involvement in decision making/management (the more involvement, the better the outcome).

What is the most appropriate base for the co-operative?

• Clinical, office and domestic facilities should be acceptable to members.
• Premises should be conveniently/equitably located for the patient populations covered.
• Scope for working alongside existing services should be explored.

What mix of in-house and contracted support services will be most appropriate?
- Size of membership, area and number of centres constrain choices.
- The level of financial support available constrains choices.
- Members may not always agree on what is essential and what optional.
- Some support from fellow tenants may be negotiable.

How will patients be informed and involved?
- Allaying the fears of patients, especially concerning home visits, reduces antagonism.
- Involving patients in planning may change attitudes.
- Discussion with CHCs is valuable.

What links can be forged with existing GP and other provider networks?
- How does the co-operative 'map' onto existing primary care groups?
- How might it relate to/work with NHS Direct?
- What are the possibilities for collaboration with other professionals providing 24-hour emergency services?

How does this model integrate or conflict with other models of care?

Theoretically, there is no reason why this model of care should not coexist and collaborate with existing, alternative methods of providing primary care outside normal surgery hours. In fact, there is considerable scope for conflict and limited examples of integration.

In areas where health authorities have chosen to use all their out-of-hours development funds to support co-operatives, general practitioners who remain outside these organisations receive no additional financial support. This applies equally to those who have chosen to maintain personal or practice rota cover and those who have no alternative. Thus, small practices covering isolated rural areas may not be welcomed by adjacent co-operatives, yet may feel that they are subsidising them. In other areas rural doctors have had some costs reimbursed, for additional receptionist time or even for out-of-hours locum assistance.

Where commercial deputising services operate in the same area as a co-operative, competition for membership may be fierce and acrimonious. In the past, there have been examples of legal challenges to co-operatives mounted by deputising services. More recently, large urban co-operatives have entered into contracts with commercial services to provide additional medical input, particularly in terms of night-time cover. Following the 1995 changes to Paragraph 13 of the GPs' terms and conditions of service, some deputising services are now also offering centre-based care.

Many co-operatives are based within or adjacent to A&E departments and minor injury units. Whilst there are examples of agreements on cross referrals and even, in at least one case, rotation of A&E nurses between co-operative triage duties and A&E department work, it is more common for each to 'defend' its territory and discourage cross referrals. The greatest level of integration appears to be within community and cottage hospitals with casualty facilities, where the GP members of the co-operative are also providing medical cover for the hospital and the lines between the two are becoming more blurred. However, the use of different funding streams is a barrier to full integration.

Co-operation with ambulance trusts is more common, but is usually restricted to a commercial transaction in which the trusts provide drivers, vehicles and message-handling services to the co-operatives.

There is more movement towards joint working with community nursing services, where on-call district nurses and community psychiatric teams may share premises with a co-operative and provide mutual assistance when necessary.

It seems that the barriers to integration are, at present, greater than the benefits.

Where is this model of care leading?

One constraint on the future development of co-operatives may be a lack of doctors who are willing to do out-of-hours work. A significant increase in doctors willing to work at night would be necessary in order to separate out-of-hours from in-hours care. The cost to member GPs would increase considerably if external doctors were employed and they were unable to defray costs with shift payments. There is also a balance to be struck between geography, demand and the number of doctors required to cope with the workload, both efficiently and with sufficient slack in the system to cope with unexpected increases in demand. There are several motivators for change. Public demand for round-the-clock access is increasing. NHS Direct will certainly have an impact, as will primary care groups and the advent of clinical governance.

Demand

The increase in demand has led to the increasing possibility of delegation. Nurses work alongside GPs in a substantial minority of co-operatives. NHS Direct will take this much further and should filter out many inappropriate calls, reducing demand on GPs by as much as 20–30%. This could take the number of telephone contacts back to the level of 1995. By triaging calls, co-operatives are already decreasing face-to-face consultations. In many co-operatives, night visits in 1998 were significantly fewer than those in preceding years.

NHS Direct

There are a number of question marks over the interface between primary care, co-operatives and NHS Direct. There is the potential for GPs to filter all their out-of-hours calls through NHS Direct, but GPs may not necessarily accept initial triage decisions made by the service. There is no reason to suppose that NHS Direct will have an impact on the viability of existing co-operatives. The Minister for Health has declared that it was the government's intention that the new service should work alongside co-operatives, allowing doctors to concentrate on medical care and enabling nurses to give advice when appropriate (NAGPC Conference, 1998).

Primary care groups

Most primary care groups (PCGs) will be smaller than the average co-operative and marginally too small for efficient out-of-hours care. This is likely to mean that one co-operative will span more than one PCG in whole or in part. This is entirely feasible. Funding streams are to be kept separate, with the out-of-hours development fund ring-fenced at health authority level for the fore-seeable future. Some PCGs may wish to commission out-of-hours care, for instance by having a primary care centre in their area. However, there may not be sufficient GPs within one area to staff it effectively and such a wish might adversely affect GPs in a neighbouring PCG. These issues will have to be resolved by negotiation. Given that co-operatives are generally highly popular with their members and that out-of-hours care has a different ethos from in-hours care, there is no reason why PCGs should significantly affect most co-operatives.

Some observers have speculated that co-operatives might take over all urgent care, both within and outside normal surgery hours. The arguments against this idea are that the clinical distinction between routine and urgent care is often not clearcut and that most GPs will want to look after their own patients in their own practices. However, others see this as a predictable next step (*see* Chapter Twelve). Home visiting out of hours has fallen, as indeed has home visiting in surgery hours, but it is unlikely to disappear completely unless the style and traditions of general practice change beyond recognition. GPs who provided out-of-hours care in a practice rota were always less likely to visit than the commercial deputising services, whose inability to respond other than by offering a home visit led to the growth of the 'visit on demand' culture among patients.

The likelihood is that PCGs will work alongside co-operatives who will develop relationships with NHS Direct that should in the end be mutually beneficial. It is possible that closer working with secondary care services might develop, notwithstanding the possible confusion that exists over relative roles. This would only occur in the long term and as a consequence of significant changes in funding streams and professional behaviour.

Clinical governance

Finally, the advent of clinical governance will influence the way in which co-operatives manage themselves. The White Paper has a series of statements about quality organisations. These are likely to provide the framework for the next series of regulations about in-house co-operative control. Coupled with the National Institution of Clinical Excellence and the growing interest in protocol-driven care, clinical governance may well produce more cost-effective and standardised treatment for out-of-hours general practice. However, it can only go so far. GPs will remain independent and will continue to show significant variation in the way in which they choose to handle particular emergencies.

References

1   Hallam L (1994) Primary medical care outside normal working hours: review of published work. *BMJ.* **308**: 249–53.

2   Department of Health and Social Security (1987) *General Medical Practitioner Workload: a report prepared for the Doctors and Dentists Review Body, 1985/86.* HMSO, London.

3   Hallam L, Cragg D (1994) Organisation of primary care services outside normal working hours. *BMJ.* **309**: 1621–3.

4   Electoral Reform Ballot Services (1992) *Your Choices for the Future: a survey of GP opinion, UK report.* ERBS, London.

5   Hallam L, Henthorne K (1998) *GP Co-operatives and Primary Care Emergency Centres: organisation and impact.* National Primary Care Research and Development Centre, Manchester.

6   Jessopp L, Beck I, Hollins L *et al.* (1997) Changing the pattern of out of hours: a survey of general practice co-operatives. *BMJ.* **314**: 199–200.

7   Bain J, Gerrard L, Russell A *et al.* (1997) The Dundee out-of-hours co-operative: preliminary outcomes for the first year of operation. *Brit J Gen Pract.* **47**: 573–4.

8   Cragg DK, Campbell SM, Roland MO (1994) Out of hours primary care centres: characteristics of those attending and declining to attend. *BMJ.* **42**: 90–1.

9   Salisbury C (1997) Observational study of a general practice out of hours co-operative: measures of activity. *BMJ.* **314**: 182–6.

10   Hallam L, Henthorne K (1999) *Providing Out-of-hours Primary Care in Northumberland.* National Primary Care Research and Development Centre, Manchester.

11   South Wiltshire Out of Hours Project (SWOOP) Group (1997) Nurse telephone triage in out of hours primary care: a pilot study. *BMJ.* **314**: 198–9.

12   Lattimer V, George S, Thompson F *et al.* (1998) Safety and effectiveness of nurse telephone consultation in out of hours primary care: randomised controlled trial. *BMJ.* **317**: 1054–9.

13   Bollam MJ, McCarthy M, Modell M (1988) Patients' assessments of out-of-hours care in general practice. *BMJ.* **296**: 829–32.

14   Sawyer L, Arber S (1982) Changes in home visiting and night and weekend cover: the patient's view. *BMJ.* **284**: 1531–4.

15   Allen D, Leavey R, Marks B (1988) Survey of patients' satisfaction with access to general practitioners. *J R Coll Gen Pract.* **38**: 163–5.

16   Salisbury C (1997) Postal survey of patients' satisfaction with a general practice out of hours cooperative. *BMJ.* **314**: 1594–8.

17   Dixon RA, Williams BT (1988) Patient satisfaction with general practitioner deputising services. *BMJ.* **297**: 1519–22.

18   Department of Health and Social Security (1984) *General Practitioner Deputising Services.* DHSS, London (Health Circular FP84).

19   Cragg D, Hallam L (1994) Quality standards for deputising services. *BMJ.* **309**: 1630.

CHAPTER SIX

GPs in A&E departments

Jeremy Dale

The challenges faced by out-of-hours general practice and accident and emergency (A&E) services have much in common. Each has experienced increasing demand over many years and involves large numbers of patients presenting with any of a vast range of problems including some that may be life threatening. They each perform vital triage and gatekeeping roles, so helping patients and the health service as a whole avoid the costs and consequences associated with unnecessary investigation and treatment. Both services need to be in a state of readiness to cope with unanticipated surges in demand, but both share persistent concerns about the appropriateness of much of their workload.

Despite these similarities, A&E services and out-of-hours services have lacked co-ordination. This lack of integration reflects long-standing differences in the way that they are commissioned, together with a history of professional mistrust and rivalries that dates back over 150 years. Before the establishment of the NHS, GPs were vehemently critical of the role casualty departments played in treating patients with general medical needs – this was seen as denying them their livelihood. Since 1948, however, there has been a tendency for GPs to distance themselves from the primary care demand that expresses itself at A&E. The system of funding GPs through capitation and items-of-service fees offered no incentives for discouraging their patients from attending A&E. Instead, GPs became increasingly concerned that any shift of demand away from A&E would lead to increased GP workload without parallel increases in resources.

From an A&E perspective, patients often appear to attend because of limitations in the availability of general practice care, particularly during out-of-hours periods. GPs are characterised as providing inadequate levels of service, leading to high rates of attendance by patients with primary care needs and stressed A&E departments with long waiting times. GPs' reluctance to see the primary care use of A&E as a problem for general practice has reinforced the negative views about general practice that pervade many A&E departments. A&E departments have been reluctant to accept primary care as a legitimate part of their work for fear of encouraging greater demand.

There has been long-standing recognition of the need to improve communication and co-operation across the A&E–primary care interface to enable better use of resources and greater continuity. However, the negative views that GPs and A&E departments hold about each other have hindered the development of more effective services. Fragmentation and poor communication between A&E and neighbouring GP services result in duplication of activity together with inconsistencies in the accessibility, availability and quality of care.

In recent years there have been some attempts to integrate aspects of A&E and general practice care, particularly in relation to the delivery of out-of-hours care. There has been evidence that when GPs gain a financial stake in A&E services, such as occurred through total purchasing pilots which gave GPs responsibility for purchasing emergency care, innovative ways of managing A&E demand are encouraged. *The New NHS* is imposing a context within which traditional professional and organisational cultures are being challenged by the drive towards partnership and integration across the health service.[1] The new commissioning arrangements give primary care groups fresh incentives to explore different ways of managing the interface between primary care and A&E services in the most cost-effective manner. The models of care that deserve consideration include GPs working in A&E departments as primary care physicians and co-ops siting their out-of-hours bases alongside or within departments. In this chapter, examples of these developments will be considered, together with issues that may influence their successful implementation.

Primary care demand at A&E

In the UK, the role of the GP as the sole provider of general medical care has never been fully accepted and A&E departments continue to be used for a wide range of non-urgent needs. Until 1948, when the NHS was established, casualty departments were the main providers of care for the poor. This led to a tradition of self-referral, especially in inner-city areas where the use of A&E services has always been strongest and general practice has tended to be less well developed. This has persisted, particularly in out-of-hours periods when access to GPs is inevitably more limited. A workload survey conducted over the 1997 Easter Bank Holiday weekend in three inner city London boroughs, for example, found that approximately 50% of primary care contacts within the area had occurred at A&E departments.[2]

Within most communities the local A&E department is seen as a key amenity, epitomising much of what the NHS is valued for: free and immediate health care. Its round-the-clock availability, on-site access to a broad range of technological facilities and expertise and direct links with outpatient clinics and admissions all contribute to its value. However, patients presenting with serious injuries or conditions that require immediate care or emergency admission comprise only a minority, generally around 15–20% of attenders. Less than 0.1% present with severe multisystem injuries. In many departments, the majority present with problems that could have been managed in a typical general practice surgery.

Rates of attendance at A&E departments have persistently been on the increase, despite universal access to general practice. It may seem self-evident that practice organisational arrangements, such as appointment systems and surgery times, influence both self-referral rates to A&E departments and out-of-hours demand. Indeed, many patients give as their reason for attending A&E lack of access to GP care. However, patterns of demand are not straightforward, reflecting the complexity involved in deciding when and where to seek help. Help-seeking behaviour is influenced not just by the structure and organisation of health services, but by much more deep-rooted societal factors. The public's expectations of the health service have increased dramatically over the years and in an increasingly consumerist society, an ever higher value is placed on the convenience and immediacy of care.

Perceptions about the appropriateness of attending A&E reflect a range of factors. Overall, the most important determinants of self-referral to A&E include:

- the person's situation when the need arises
- the perceived availability and accessibility of A&E and GP services
- the patient or an adviser's view of urgency and the type of care that is required
- perceptions of the costs and benefits involved in attending A&E or general practice.

The decision to seek care often reflects a social process, influenced by lay people and the advice they give. In addition to family, friends and neighbours, other 'lay' referrers, such as teachers, employers, policemen and passers-by, may all be involved in the decision making, although they may lack knowledge about the patient's GP's arrangements. They may therefore be more inclined to suggest that the patient attends an A&E department. It is not surprising that efforts to educate patients to make more 'appropriate' use of out-of-hours or A&E services have been largely ineffectual.

A&E services are usually depicted as being overburdened – crowded departments, lengthy waiting times and stressed staff – but there are concerns about the appropriateness of much of the care that is provided. Indeed, there are several reasons for supposing that A&E care may be less effective for patients with primary care or non-urgent problems than care provided by GPs. A&E staff are highly trained in the diagnostic and technical skills appropriate to life-saving and acute trauma care, but often lack the interest and skills necessary for effectively meeting primary care needs. As a result, patients with such needs may receive care that is both inappropriate and costly. Important clinical matters may be overlooked and there may be unnecessary duplication of activities and procedures, but such care may confirm in the patient's mind the validity of their fears and so increase their anxiety and perception of threat. A&E staff generally have limited knowledge about local primary care health services and may lack confidence in them. This may deter them from referring patients back to general practice. For the patient, it may contribute to raising expectations for high-technology medicine and so encourage future dependency on hospital services.

Many factors are now driving change at the A&E–primary care interface. In addition to increasing emphasis on cost effectiveness and service quality across the whole of the health service, those most relevant to the development of out-of-hours services include:

- increased recognition of the overlap between services provided by A&E and GP departments
- shift from home visiting to base attendance in out-of-hours care
- potential economies of scale from siting out-of-hours bases alongside or within A&E departments
- increased recognition of the role GPs can play as gatekeepers at A&E and concerns about the appropriateness of care provided by A&E department staff
- new unified commissioning arrangements.

The site chosen for an out-of-hours GP centre is likely to have workload, quality of care and financial implications and may have an appreciable influence on A&E department workload. There is some evidence that patients prefer to attend out-of-hours centres sited near or alongside A&E departments, rather than at sites outside the hospital. In 1995, 20 co-ops were contacted to investigate their choice of where to site out-of-hours centres.[3] The co-ops ranged in size: the smallest with 47 GPs serving a rural setting to the largest with 230 GPs serving an urban population of almost half a million. Two of the co-ops had bases in A&E departments or minor injury units. They reported that 50% and 66% of their callers attended the centre. Eight co-ops had bases in cottage/community hospitals, some of which had separate minor injury unit facilities. The proportion of their callers who agreed to attend the centres varied from 4% (for an inner city co-op) to 45% (for a suburban co-op). Ten co-ops were based in community settings which varied from health clinics, a fire station and an airport building to an office along-side a motorway junction. Between 7% and 37% of their callers attended a base. Those co-ops that had bases on hospital premises achieved higher rates of patient attendance at the base than those in community settings and the highest levels of all were achieved in those that were based alongside A&E or minor injury unit departments.

A variety of interventions have been tried or suggested as means of managing the demand at A&E. Some have been aimed at limiting access, such as giving triage nurses the authority to turn patients away from A&E. These, though, face ethical, legal and clinical objections, particularly in relation to the needs of socially deprived populations who may have limited access to other sources of care. GPs also object because of fears that such obstacles will merely redirect workload towards themselves, so placing additional strain on within-hours and out-of-hours services.

The attention being given to improving the quality of care across the primary–secondary care interface has meant that policymakers, planners and purchasers have become more interested in identifying new ways of responding to the demand for primary care at A&E and in setting standards for such services. There has been increasing recognition of the need to do this within the context of planning integrated emergency care systems. There is a need for consistency in the care provided by different providers if demand is to be effectively and appropriately managed.

For at least 25 years, there has been interest in developing more primary care-oriented responses at A&E. In 1974, the House of Commons Expenditure Committee suggested that consideration should be given to making available, particularly in large city A&E departments, an emergency general practice service staffed by GPs on a rota basis. This was reflected by the 1978 Royal Commission on the National Health Service[4] which stated that 'where the tradition of using [A&E as a walk-in GP surgery] is strong, it may be preferable for the hospital to accept this role and make specific arrangements for fulfilling it, rather than to try and resist established local preferences'.

The approaches used by GPs to problem solve, elicit patients' needs, cope with diagnostic uncertainty and risk taking and ensure continuity of care all appear to be highly relevant to managing primary care needs within an A&E setting. GPs have more experience than hospital doctors in managing the broad variety of presentations seen in primary care and more highly developed consultation skills. They are more likely to use time as a deliberate diagnostic aid and to identify, understand and treat patients' needs within a broader psychosocial context. They will be more familiar with the availability of local health services and how to make best use of them. They are likely to have greater skill at defining the appropriate level of care that is required and so are better able to advise about self-care and to negotiate appropriate follow-up with the patient.

Integrating care across the A&E–primary care interface not only creates opportunities for providing more appropriate care for the needs of existing A&E users, but it also may support the provision of more effective and efficient out-of-hours services by GPs. Box 6.1 summarises the case for employing GPs in the A&E department to treat patients attending with primary care needs from the perspective of improving A&E services. Box 6.2 outlines the case from the perspective of co-ops and deputising services for siting out-of-hours consulting bases within or alongside A&E departments. From society's perspective, providing non-urgent care at A&E may be an efficient use of healthcare resources, particularly for people who have difficulty attending GP services during normal working hours.

Box 6.1: Assumptions underlying the employment of Primary Care Physicians in A&E

- Patients often present at A&E with vague, undifferentiated problems.
- The stressful and hectic environment that characterises A&E departments makes patient-focused care difficult to provide.
- Few medical or nursing staff in A&E have received training in appropriate consultation skills for managing patients with primary care problems.
- GPs are more experienced than junior A&E staff at managing a broad variety of presentations and have been trained to assess the relative importance of symptoms and signs at early stages of illness, to cope with diagnostic uncertainty and so define the appropriate level of care that is required.
- GPs are more effective gatekeepers in A&E than hospital staff, make more appropriate use of resources and provide more cost-effective care.
- GPs are familiar with the health services available in their local community, including how to refer to them and make best use of them, and so encourage greater continuity of care.
- Employing GPs in A&E encourages greater understanding about primary care throughout the department and so contributes to challenging some of the negative views that staff in A&E departments traditionally hold.
- Working in A&E may add to GPs' job satisfaction, provide new challenges and opportunities for self-development and lessen professional isolation.

> **Box 6.2:** Arguments given by co-op managers for siting centres within or
> near an A&E department
>
> - The acceptability to patients, with ease of parking and security.
> - Familiarity of location to local community.
> - Usually accessible by public or private transport and in most areas well
>   signposted.
> - Increased credibility in the eyes of the local community from being closely
>   linked to the hospital.
> - 'One-stop' care – whether the patient requires advice, an investigation,
>   referral to an on-call team or admission.
> - Improved communication and relationships between local GPs and hospital
>   colleagues, making referral to hospital colleagues more straightforward.
> - Potential cost savings – hospital could provide ancillary maintenance and
>   support staff for the base (including portering, security and reception staff
>   if required).
> - In some areas where GPs have access to their own inpatient beds, siting an
>   out-of-hours centre within the hospital site may enable ease of cover.
> - Potential opportunity for income generation, such as through negotiating
>   a contract to provide primary care services to the A&E department.
> - Shared opportunities between GPs and hospital colleagues for training sup-
>   port and development around clinical issues, administration and manage-
>   ment of out-of-hours services for co-op members and staff.
> - Attractive to service commissioners and hospital trusts, might lead to more
>   seamless services and more efficient use of both primary care and hospital
>   resources.

The case study below gives a detailed account of the benefits identified by the
evaluation of the A&E primary care service at King's College Hospital,
London.[5,6]

CASE STUDY OF AN EXAMPLE OF GOOD PRACTICE

The model of A&E primary care developed at King's College Hospital
provides an example of how greater partnership and integration of A&E
and general practice care can lead to improved effectiveness. Recruiting
GPs as clinical assistants and expanding the roles of nurses is not a new
means of coping with the difficulties experienced by many A&E departments. In the early 1950s, for example, the General Medical Services
Committee of the BMA recommended that help for the casualty department from local GPs should be encouraged because of the shortage of

junior hospital doctors. However, until the project initiated at King's, GPs had not been recruited to work in A&E departments specifically for their primary care expertise.

King's is a teaching hospital in an inner-city area in south-east London characterised by high levels of social deprivation. Since 1989, GPs have been employed in the department on a sessional basis as primary care physicians. The service was initiated within a research project to test its clinical and cost effectiveness. The project resulted from collaboration between the medical school's Department of General Practice Studies and the hospital's Department of A&E Medicine, together with the support of the district health authority, the family health services authority (then the family practitioner committee) and the local medical committee. It reflected the A&E department's philosophy of care which was that any patient who chooses to attend the department should be treated as a legitimate user of the service. The local support for the project reflected work to improve care across the primary–secondary care interface that the A&E consultant and the head of the Department of General Practice Studies had been involved in over many years. This contributed to engendering trust and understanding between GPs and staff at the A&E department.

Employing GPs in A&E was intended as a means of providing more responsive and appropriate care. The aim was to respond to each patient's immediate healthcare needs with the minimum of intervention, whenever appropriate redirecting the patient back to community-based primary care services for further care and follow-up.

The first steps involved in setting up the service were to designate a consulting room in the A&E department as a 'primary care surgery', to adapt the triage system to provide a means for prospectively identifying the primary care content of patients' presentations based on perceived need for care (Box 6.3) and to recruit GP principals from the local area

---

Box 6.3:   Triage criteria for 'primary care' and 'A&E' attenders

'Primary care' attenders
- Self-referred patients with conditions not in need of immediate resuscitation or urgent care and unlikely to require hospital admission
- Self-referred patients with non-urgent complications of chronic conditions

'A&E' attenders
- All patients referred by letter or phone by a GP
- All emergency presentations in need of immediate care or likely to require admission
- Trauma requiring urgent hospital assessment (e.g. clinically fractured bones and dislocations, head injuries with loss of consciousness)

to work on a sessional basis as A&E primary care physicians. Originally, six GPs were employed, but since 1992 there have been between ten and 14 GPs employed at any one time, each working one or two 3–4-hour sessions per week. The current rates of pay are £30–35 per hour depending on the time of day and day of the week. The criterion for appointment is that the doctor should have undergone full vocational training and be committed to the aims of the service, and preference is given to those with previous A&E experience and interest in team work.

Nurses performing triage have at least six months experience of the A&E department and undergo training which includes practical supervision and learning about the expertise and skills of local general practitioners. Applying the triage criteria at King's has resulted in around 40% of attenders being categorised as 'primary care', a proportion that has persisted over the last decade.

Since 1992, the service has been commissioned as part of the A&E department contract. Most sessions occur outside GPs' normal consulting hours: early afternoon, evening and at weekends. GPs see approximately 8000 patients per year and by 1998, had accumulated a total of approximately 50 000 patients.

The service was initially evaluated as part of a controlled prospective trial involving six GPs, 27 senior house officers (SHOs), four registrars and 4641 patients attending with primary care needs.[5,6] This demonstrated consistent differences between the GPs and the A&E doctors in rates of investigations, treatments and referrals for patients with primary care problems. For example, compared to the GPs, SHOs ordered X-rays more than twice as frequently and ordered blood tests around six times as often. Referrals to hospital outpatient clinics or on-call teams occurred almost three times as frequently. This greater level of intervention did not appear to influence clinical outcome or patient satisfaction and the yield of clinically important findings appeared to be similar for all groups. GPs appeared to encourage patients to become less dependent on hospital-based care and instead encouraged confidence in and use of community-based teams.

The analysis of average costs (excluding A&E department capital costs and overheads) indicated a potential saving of £61 000 per year at 1991 prices if GPs, SHOs and registrars treated the same proportions of the primary care workload over the duration of a year as they did in the study sample (that is, the GPs treat just over a third of the 'primary care' workload, approximately 8300 patients per year). If the costs of differences observed in subsequent rates of admission were included, this figure increased to around £150 000 per annum.

In summary, this case study indicates how employing GPs within the A&E department may lead to more effective use of available human and capital resources, contributing to immediate and potential longer term benefits for patients and the health service. The experience and problem-solving strategies employed by GPs appeared to enable a greater proportion of patients to be seen without resorting to investigations, referrals and other costly interventions. GPs reported that working in A&E led to overall increased job satisfaction and greater variation in their pattern of work and opportunities for professional development (minor surgery, treatment room care, etc.).

Employing GPs in A&E appeared to be a highly effective way of challenging attitudes through the skills and knowledge that they directly bring into the department. The familiarity and understanding resulting from closer working may lead to more effective communication between community- and hospital-based teams and may reinforce future use of community-based services. It also supports the development of stronger links between GPs who would not otherwise work together.

A&E staff felt that employing GPs had resulted in reduced levels of stress for all staff, improved patient satisfaction and reduced complaints. They felt that it also allowed more time for A&E doctors to manage patients with urgent, life-threatening needs. They felt that the improved level of care and staff morale within the department helped the recruitment and retention of high-quality nursing and medical staff.

Since completing the research project, there has been continuous audit of investigations, referrals and prescriptions. This has confirmed that the pattern of care and levels of intervention observed during the study have persisted. Patient satisfaction has remained high. There have been very few complaints received during this period relating to clinical care of patients treated in A&E by GPs.

More recently, the local out-of-hours co-operative has been negotiating a contract whereby patients who require face-to-face consultation can be referred to the A&E primary care service to see a GP working a session in the department. This might reduce the workload on GPs working sessions for the co-operative, while making more effective use of the GP based in the A&E department. It could enable the co-operative to offer patients the opportunity of attending a GP based at a site that may be more accessible to the patient than the co-operative's main out-of-hours centre and so may help reduce the home visiting rate.

Evidence from other evaluations

Evidence supporting the applicability of the King's model of A&E primary care to other sites has emerged from a number of studies in the UK and Ireland. Murphy *et al.* studied five GPs employed in the A&E department of St James's Hospital, Dublin, on a sessional basis to manage patients triaged as 'non-urgent' (66% of all new attenders) and compared these GPs' consultations to those of 34 usual A&E medical staff.[7] In all, 4684 patients were studied and the findings confirmed lower GP use of diagnostic investigations and fewer referrals to outpatient and inpatient services. GPs referred more patients back to general practice for follow-up. No differences were found in outcome measures (health status and patient satisfaction) between patients seen by the different types of doctor.

Ward *et al.* studied 1078 patients triaged as presenting with primary care problems at St Mary's Hospital, London.[8] According to workload and whether or not a GP was on duty, 58.4% of these patients had been seen by GPs employed on a sessional basis and the remainder saw A&E staff. In total, ten GPs were included in the study, which again confirmed that GPs made lower use of investigations and made fewer referrals to on-call teams and outpatient clinics. All staff involved had positive perceptions of the scheme.

Following commendation of the King's A&E primary care service by the National Audit Office[9] and the Tomlinson Inquiry,[10] several A&E departments in London established similar initiatives. As a result, considerable investment took place across London in establishing schemes similar to the King's A&E primary care service. By 1995, around £900 000 per annum out of primary care development funds (1% of the London Initiative Zone budget) was being invested in such services.

From the evaluations of the A&E primary care developments in west and south-east London,[11] these initiatives appeared to be highly valued and supported by local purchasers and patient and GP representatives. While some districts have experienced difficulty recruiting adequate numbers of appropriately qualified GPs to work as A&E primary care physicians, where they have been successful, the GPs working within such schemes identify considerable personal and professional benefits. These include increased diversity and challenge in their working week from working with a different population of patients as part of a different team of doctors and nurses. In addition, the educational benefits of working within A&E are perceived to be valuable. The effectiveness of developments based on the King's model rests on the quality of triage nurse assessments, and staff training and audit is of crucial importance to ensure that primary care patients are identified in a consistent and reliable manner.

A number of variants to the King's model of A&E primary care have also emerged. One that has been implemented in at least three London A&E departments is the employment of a vocationally trained GP as a full-time A&E primary care consultant to lead primary care service developments, including the primary care training of medical and nursing staff. Such consultants may form important points of liaison between primary care and hospital services, but the direct impact of these appointments on the quality of care provided to patients has not been formally evaluated.

In some departments, there has been interest in developing nurse practitioner roles in preference to employing GPs within A&E. While much has been written in the UK about the work of nurse practitioners, there has been little evaluation of their role in terms of cost effectiveness. Nurse practitioners are not necessarily cheaper to employ than doctors; it costs about 25% more per hour to employ a 'G' grade nurse than a SHO and they usually see fewer patients per hour. Although nurse practitioners are cheaper to employ than GPs, as was found in west London the differences in the rate at which patients are assessed and treated by nurse practitioners and GPs can result in nurse practitioner care being more costly overall. In general, nurse practitioners tend to manage a narrower range of presenting problems than A&E doctors and their caseloads contain more trauma. 10–15% or more of A&E patients can be treated by a nurse practitioner, depending on the scope of the nurses' training and local guidelines and protocols. However, the improved communication across the A&E–primary care interface and other gains that appear to follow from employing local GPs in A&E may not be observed.

Issues to consider in planning new service developments

In this chapter we have seen that employing GPs in A&E departments offers ways of integrating the provision of A&E services and out-of-hours GP services. It can enable more consistent care across the A&E–primary care interface and more cost-effective use of health service resources, and may reduce waiting times. While the commissioning arrangements being introduced within the health service reforms provide primary care groups with new incentives to consider such models of care, the applicability of specific A&E primary care developments to any one area will depend upon a range of local factors. These include:

- the geography and sociodemographic characteristics of the catchment population

- the volume and case mix of the A&E department and the out-of-hours services
- the support of key stakeholders within the health authority, the hospital trust and general practice
- the availability of adequate resources to meet the needs of new service developments.

The primary care workload in many A&E departments is insufficient to make the employment of GPs as A&E primary care physicians a cost-effective option unless linked into the overall organisational arrangements for managing out-of-hours care within the district. The King's model is likely to have greatest relevance to large, inner-city departments serving commuting, tourist and/or socially deprived and homeless populations, but in other areas there may be opportunities for developing hybrids of the King's model. For example, one GP co-operative in South London negotiated an annual contract in 1995 to treat up to 10 000 A&E patients. Following assessment by a triage nurse, patients attending with primary care needs are referred from the A&E department to the co-op where they are treated by the doctor doing base sessions. Such developments may be restrained by features of the local geography and services, such as where the local hospital with an A&E department is relatively inaccessible or lacks suitable space for an out-of-hours centre.

Attitudes of healthcare professionals

The main obstacle to developing more integrated services is usually the attitudes of healthcare professionals and managers. In areas which lack a history of collaboration around the A&E–primary care interface, developing more integrated care between A&E and general practice may be an uphill struggle. As we have seen, the culture and philosophies of care of general practice and A&E departments have traditionally been at odds. Such views are likely to have inextricable links with the history, structures, personalities and relationships between individuals and professional groups within any district. Staff within A&E departments tend to be hostile to both the demand for primary care at A&E and general practice as a whole. In many areas, A&E consultants are still very resistant to accepting primary care as a legitimate part of their remit or recognising the role that GPs could play within their departments. A&E consultants often express the concern that providing more responsive care to patients attending with primary care needs could 'open the floodgates' to demand. This, though, does not seem to have been the experience in districts where out-of-hours services have sited their centres within or near to A&E departments or where GPs are employed in A&E as primary care physicians.

GPs tend to be wary of the potential implications for their responsibilities and workload of developing closer links with A&E departments and many are resistant to the idea of siting out-of-hours centres within or near A&E. For many, A&E work is an anathema; avoidance of the hospital environment and its structures is part of what attracted them into general practice. Many fear that demand might become more difficult to control at out-of-hours centres sited near to an A&E department, as this might encourage a 'walk-in' mentality among patients, with GPs increasingly compelled to see A&E patients. GPs often anticipate that the A&E consultants at their local hospital will be unenthusiastic about siting the out-of-hours centre near their department and so expect that it will be difficult to negotiate satisfactory arrangements.

Successfully implementing service developments at the A&E–primary care interface involves creating a receptive local environment. The process of achieving shared ownership and support for the purpose and goals of new service developments has resource implications. The strengths and weaknesses of different options will need to be considered and the extent to which each meets local requirements. The experience from districts that have established A&E–primary care services is that the way that ideas and information are presented and disseminated may be critical. It has been demonstrated in several areas that through investing in communication and dialogue with key individuals and groups, it is possible to overcome the resistance imposed by traditional organisational values and constraints.

New training programmes may be needed for both A&E staff and GPs about how best to work together. At King's College Hospital, for example, programmes that have been implemented include weekly primary care skills training for SHOs and an A&E nurse–practice nurse exchange scheme.[12] Orientation and induction procedures for GPs working within A&E departments, guidelines and ongoing audit are essential to maintain the consistency and quality of the service.

As with any process of change management, the enthusiasm of key individuals will determine the extent to which organisational and cultural constraints and the competing interests of different professional groups and their members are overcome. Without effective leadership, management, staff development and training, new services will not run efficiently and the potential benefits of closer working between GPs and A&E departments are unlikely to be realised.

References

1 Department of Health (1997) *The New NHS: Modern, Dependable.* HMSO, London.

2 Hollins L (1997) *A 'Snapshot' of Out of Hours and Emergency Services in Lambeth, Southwark and Lewisham Health Authority.* LSL Out of Hours Project, King's College School of Medicine and Dentistry, London.

3 Dale J (1996) Where to site an emergency centre. *Management Gen Pract.* **19**: 16–19.

4 Royal Commission's Report on the NHS (1978) *Chapter 10: accident and emergency services.* HMSO, London.

5 Dale J, Green J, Reid F, Glucksman E, Higgs R (1995) Primary care in the accident and emergency department: II. Comparison of general practitioners and hospital doctors. *BMJ.* **311**: 427–30.

6 Dale J, Lang H, Roberts J, Green J, Glucksman E (1996) Cost effectiveness of treating primary care patients in accident and emergency: a comparison between general practitioners, senior house officers and registrars. *BMJ.* **312**: 1340–4.

7 Murphy AW, Bury G, Plunkett PK *et al.* (1996) Randomised controlled trial of general practitioner versus usual medical care in an urban accident and emergency department: process, outcome, and comparative cost. *BMJ.* **312**: 1135–42.

8 Ward P, Huddy J, Hargreaves S *et al.* (1996) Primary care in London: an evaluation of general practitioners working in an inner city accident and emergency department. *J Accident Emerg Med.* **13**: 11–15.

9 National Audit Office (1992) *Report of the Controller and Auditor General. NHS Accident and Emergency Departments in England.* HMSO, London.

10 Tomlinson Inquiry (1992) *Report of the Inquiry into London's Health Service, Medical Education and Research.* HMSO, London.

11 Dale J, Dolan B, Morley V (1996) Take five. *Health Service J.* **16 May**: 30–1.

12 Crouch R, Dale J, Haverty S, Winsor S (1996) Piloting an A&E and practice nurse educational exchange. *Br J Nursing.* **5**(22): 1387–90.

CHAPTER SEVEN

Nurse telephone consultation

Valerie Lattimer and Robert Crouch

Telephone consultation is an increasingly important component of healthcare. In this chapter, we outline the development of nurse telephone consultation in out-of-hours primary care, present two organisational models as examples of good practice and discuss evidence about safety, effectiveness and acceptability. We offer some practical suggestions for setting up telephone consultation services and we consider possible future developments in the context of the national implementation of NHS Direct.

The percentage of households in Britain with a telephone rose from 42% in 1972 to 94% in 1997.[1] In addition, there has been a dramatic growth in the use of mobile phones. The phone is an increasingly essential part of everyday life and services such as banking, insurance and shopping are increasingly accessed by telephone.

We use the term 'telephone consultation' to refer to the process by which healthcare professionals, usually doctors or nurses, assess and manage calls from patients or their carers about health-related problems. Calls may be managed by offering information and advice or by referral for a face-to-face consultation or to another health or social care agency.

Although many nurses routinely have contact with patients over the telephone, few have been specifically trained for this role. Until recently there was limited interest in developing the telephone consultation skills of healthcare professionals. However, it has now become an important and mainstream part of primary care. Many general practices, for example, have dedicated 'phone-in' periods for patients and use telephone consultation as a means of screening requests for same-day appointments. Practice nurses, health visitors and district nurses also make substantial use of the telephone in their routine contact with patients.

In the wider context, a broad range of helpline services provides information and support to individuals, carers and their families. Examples include Macmillan Cancer Relief, Saneline and Samaritans in the voluntary sector, as well as NHS Direct and the NHS regional health information services. A valuable role is also played by community pharmacists. They often deal with requests for advice about medication and minor illness over the phone. In hospitals, telephone consultation is used for patient follow-up and, increasingly, for linking healthcare professionals in remote sites to major centres.

The overall shift that has taken place in recent years towards providing telephone advice during out-of-hours periods has been discussed in earlier parts of this book and so will not be considered in detail here. Three key factors appear to have contributed to the development of telephone consultation in out-of-hours primary care: rising demand; changing patterns of work and approaches to care, with increasing use of information and communications technology; and the growing acceptability of telephone services. Around a third of co-operatives and many deputising services now employ nurses to provide telephone consultations.

The evidence base for nurse telephone consultation

Until recently there has been little evidence about the effectiveness, safety and acceptability of telephone consultation. Few studies have been undertaken in real rather than simulated situations and few have been comparative. Outcomes have not always been well defined and data collection periods have usually been very brief (often less than one month).[2] Most of the literature emanates from outside the UK and so may not be applicable to the circumstances within the NHS. Although nurse telephone consultation is well established in other healthcare systems, rigorous trials to test the safety and effectiveness appear not to have been undertaken.

A recent review[3] found several examples of serious inadequacies in telephone consultations.[4-6] Sometimes the most obvious questions, such as the age of the patient, were not asked before advice is given. A particular problem seems to relate to decisions being made about what is wrong with the patient and their needs before an adequate history has been obtained, aptly described in one paper as the phenomenon of 'the mind snapping shut'.[7] Concerns remain about the accuracy and reliability of assessment and advice given to callers.[8] Two recent evaluations of nurse telephone consultation in the UK,[9,10] however, provide reassuring evidence in its support. The services that they relate to and their main findings are discussed below.

Telephone consultation – nurse-led models for primary care

Two out-of-hours primary care services in which nurses play a key role are WILCODOC and HARMONI. Both services have more than two years experience of nurse telephone consultation, have developed elaborate organisational processes for the employment and professional development of their staff and use the Telephone Advice System (TAS),[3] a password-protected computer-based decision support program that is linked to each co-operative's administrative software. Both services have been the subject of robust evaluations.

WILCODOC was formed in March 1996 with 55 members and a registered patient population of 97 000. The co-operative covers two zones: the city of Salisbury and the more rural Salisbury Plain. It commenced nurse telephone consultation in January 1997. Two GPs and two nurses are on duty and two GPs are on standby to assist if necessary, throughout evenings and weekends. In all, 13 nurses are employed with primary care experience in practice nursing, health visiting, district nursing and A&E nursing. A senior nurse leads and supervises the team. Most of the nurses retain other part-time posts in the NHS. This has been encouraged as one way in which the nurses can retain direct patient contact.

HARMONI (Harrow Medics Out of Hours Network Inc) was established in 1996 with 120 GP members. The service is based in west London and covers a socially mixed, multiethnic population. It has rapidly grown in size and scale and by 1999 included over 430 GPs covering a population of 1 million people. From its inception, nurses were employed to provide a telephone consultation service including call triage and prioritisation of calls for GP visits. By the end of 1998, nurses had completed over 200 000 telephone consultations. The service has now expanded further to become part of a second-wave NHS Direct pilot.

HARMONI employs 56 nurses with experience in community, A&E or primary care nursing on a sessional basis (the number of sessions undertaken by the nurses varies from three to eight per month).

Developing the organisation

The efficiency and effectiveness of nurse telephone consultation, like any other service, rests on the way that it is implemented and managed and this is likely to involve considerable investment in organisational development and infrastructure. This includes equipping the call centre offices, including telephone and computer networks, and recruiting and training staff. This inevitably is a costly process. In addition, new management systems have to be set up for the nurses and policies and procedures have to be agreed and implemented relating to not only clinical aspects of the service but also employment aspects including health and safety of employees. Contingency plans have to be made and rehearsed for such eventualities as system failures or overload.

The pathway of care

The pathway of care is similar at WILCODOC and HARMONI. Callers speak first to a receptionist who checks and inputs the patient's name, age and location and then transfers the caller to one of the nurses on duty. If no nurse is available, the receptionist asks the caller whether they consider the situation to be an emergency and if not, agree that the nurse will call back.

On commencing the clinical assessment, the nurse has the patient's details on screen, together with a summary of any calls previously assessed using TAS. The nurse elicits the patient's symptoms and history using the TAS guidelines and, according to the needs identified, offers standardised advice or refers the patient for a consultation at one of the out-of-hours surgeries or arranges a home visit .

If in doubt about how best to manage the situation, nurses can refer the call to a GP. Callers can also request to speak to a GP if they require further information or reassurance. Callers are always advised not to hesitate to call back if they are concerned or if the patient's condition worsens. In some situations the caller may be asked to ring back after an agreed interval to let the nurse know of progress. Nurses can also use the diary facility in TAS to automatically remind them to return a call at a particular time.

At WILCODOC, at the end of a period of duty and ideally during the shift, nurses contact the GP on duty to report back on the calls they have managed. They also work closely with the receptionist to ensure that all calls and the outcome of calls can be accounted for.

Preparatory and continuing professional education

Education and training are key to developing a safe and reliable service and the learning needs of different staff may have to be addressed: for example, nurse advisers; senior nurses with supervisory responsibilities; call handlers or receptionists. Box 7.1 sets out suggested learning outcomes for inclusion in an education programme. Nurses initially learn about the knowledge and skills involved in telephone consultation and receive training in the use of decision support software, prior to a period of supervised practice.

Box 7.1: Examples of learning outcomes for nurse telephone consultation skills training

- Know the aims, core values and scope of the service.
- Demonstrate unconditional positive regard for callers and a non-judgemental approach to care which avoids stereotyping.
- Communicate effectively in time-limited situations by quickly establishing trust, using listening, questioning and negotiating and information-giving skills; checking caller understanding and inviting call back.
- Undertake systematic patient assessment by identifying caller concerns and expectations; talking directly to the patient where possible; eliciting a clinical history; building a picture of the situation; negotiating the nature of the problem; checking that nothing more serious could be happening and making a triage decision.
- Make appropriate and timely referrals so that the patient receives safe care in the right place at the right time.
- Manage difficult to detect and potentially life-threatening problems in adults and children. Identify and respond to medical emergencies by expediting the dispatch of emergency services; supporting and instructing callers in emergency situations and where necessary staying on the line to provide interim first aid until help arrives at the scene.
- Respond to callers who express suicidal ideation, who are threatening to harm themselves or others and make appropriate referrals to other agencies.
- State responsibilities under the Child Protection Act and in responding to calls from children.
- Understand the requirements of professional accountability, confidentiality and record keeping in the context of telephone consultation.
- Develop skills in managing 'difficult' calls such as hoax calls or sexually motivated calls.

Training in the use of decision support software is an important element as nurses generally are not familiar with using computers during consultations. There is often some fear attached to the use of information technology. Training is given at two levels: user and system administration. It is delivered in a cascade format with one or two nurses trained at the sites to a higher level to facilitate staff support and provide on-site troubleshooting.

Training in the use of the software is intended to consolidate nurses' telephone consultation skills. Learning after instruction is experiential in nature and is based on a series of case vignettes designed to draw out all the elements of effective consultation and to ensure clinical safety. Familiarisation before 'going live' usually takes a minimum of 20 hours.

The guidelines incorporated in the TAS represent a consensus view of the signs, symptoms and issues to be considered when assessing callers' clinical need and the advice that should be given. They are based on currently accepted clinical knowledge and practice, relevant literature and texts and advice from relevant specialists. The TAS guidelines are age and sex specific. The question structure is designed to highlight areas that should be considered but may not appear immediately obvious given the presenting complaint. It prompts the nurse to ask 'critical questions' to ensure that urgent and potentially urgent situations are not overlooked.

Establishing competency before individuals 'go live' with consultations is fundamental. This can be achieved using case scenarios and predetermined criteria for competency in terms of both consultation skills and clinical assessment skills. The computer system provides the necessary documentation to support this process. As with any skill, repeated exposure and practice of that skill is important in maintaining competence.

By 2000, academically accredited courses in telephone consultation are likely to be more widely available. The advantage of enabling nurses to access courses validated in higher education is that completion can lead to an award with CAT points (credit accumulation and transfer) which may form part of a pathway to a degree. Investing in staff development may be an important aspect of staff retention.

Quality assurance

A variety of approaches to audit and quality improvement have been developed. It is essential that these are systematised so that quality assurance becomes a routine and ongoing process. TAS automatically generates reports relating to the call length and outcomes of calls that can be used to compare the practice of individual nurses with that of their peers. These can be used to identify nurses who may be in need of further training.

Concurrent or retrospective indepth call review is possibly the best way to examine clinical practice. Apart from clearcut considerations, such as whether or not a nurse referred a call to a GP as required by the guidelines, much of what constitutes clinical excellence is a matter of judgement. Two methods of approaching indepth review may be helpful.

Calls can be usefully reviewed in detail through one-to-one clinical supervision with the senior nurse, though much can also be gained through self-assessment and peer review. The nurse is invited to select a case for review which they found 'tricky' in some respect and feel that they may not have handled well. They bring their reflections on the call, the computer or paper record and the audio-taped recording to the supervision meeting. Constructive exploration of what went well during the call and what could have been improved form the basis for discussion and learning.

Multidisciplinary case review meetings with nurses and GPs to discuss the management of particular calls or types of calls can also be used to generate points of learning which should inform the ongoing development of the service. Regular, for example bimonthly, meetings may help to foster a learning environment in which nursing staff feel valued for their contributions to the service.

Evaluation of nurse telephone consultation

Both WILCODOC and HARMONI have evaluated aspects of the quality of their services.

Triage decisions

A randomised controlled trial of the WILCODOC service included 14 492 calls received during specified times over a 12-month period: 7184 calls in the intervention arm (nurse telephone consultation) and 7308 calls in the control arm (standard GP co-operative care).[9] Nurses managed 50% of calls during intervention periods; GP telephone advice was reduced by 69%; patient attendance at an out-of-hours primary care centre was reduced by 38% and GP home visits were reduced by 23%. The ten most frequent presenting complaints were fever, vomiting, abdominal pain, cough, cold/flu, breathing difficulty, headache, rash, diarrhoea and earache.

Analysis of 10 188 calls to HARMONI taken by 25 nurses identified that the five most commonly used assessment pathways were fever, cough, cold symptoms, vomiting and headache. In terms of outcome following nurse assessment, 49.2% of the calls were advised of the need for face-to-face consultation either by home visit (15.3%), base visit (30.6%), by attending A&E (2.2%) or by calling 999 (1.1%). The remainder (50.8%) were given advice by the nurse.

Efficiency

Many potential benefits for patients and GPs have been identified from experience of operating nurse telephone consultation services, though these need to be tested in further research. GP workload can be prioritised, so that the most urgent cases are seen first. GP workload can be reduced, allowing more time to be spent with patients who are visited or who attend the base to be seen. Callers may have faster access to assessment and advice from a healthcare professional and, where patient attendances at an out-of-hours surgery are reduced, patient costs may be reduced.

The data from HARMONI give an indication of length of nurse consultations. The mean call duration (including time taken to call the patient back and complete documentation) was 6.73 minutes (SD 2.94, 95% CI 6.68–6.79). There was a mean difference of 18.6 seconds (95% CI 12.1–25.8) between calls managed by advice and those where any type of face-to-face medical consultation was recommended.

Clinical safety

Gains in efficiency are only acceptable if patient safety is maintained. The randomised controlled trial of the WILCODOC service demonstrated equivalence in the number of deaths within seven days of contact with the out-of-hours service, in emergency admissions to hospital within three days and in the number of patients attending the A&E department within three days of a contact. Nurse telephone consultation was shown to be at least as safe as standard co-operative care, though the processes of care leading to death or to admission in the study have still to be reviewed. Clearly, deaths may be expected or unexpected and emergency hospital admissions may be desirable and timely or may be an outcome of suboptimal care.

Acceptability

Evidence of the acceptability of telephone consultation in the primary care setting remains limited and further research is needed to better understand callers' expectations and experiences of telephone management.

During the trial year, WILCODOC received only two complaints concerning care given during intervention periods, one of which concerned a nurse. At HARMONI, the service has proved very acceptable to patients. During the first six months of the service, four informal complaints were received that involved nurses. There was no evidence, however, that the health of any patient had been adversely affected.

Cost implications

There are few data available about the cost effectiveness of nurse telephone consultation. In part, this reflects the difficulty of costing out-of-hours general medical services within the NHS and the value placed on GPs' time outside normal surgery hours. The establishment of a nurse telephone consultation service may incur substantial set-up costs. In large co-operatives, a nurse service may enable the number of GPs on duty at any one time to be reduced but in smaller co-operatives which require only one or two GPs on shift at any one time, this is less likely to be possible. Consideration needs to be given not only to the financial costs of different out-of-hours arrangements, but also the opportunity costs associated with them.

Accountability, liability and quality

One of the main concerns co-operatives have about employing nurses for telephone consultations relates to responsibility and liability for their decisions and the advice that is given. It is clear that the nurse is accountable to both her professional body and her employer for his/her acts or omissions during telephone consultation. Nurses are professionally accountable for all aspects of their practice (which includes telephone consultation) and if a nurse fails to perform competently they may be called before a conduct committee of the UKCC, the body that registers nurses in the UK. If a nurse gives advice or makes a decision that does not meet the legal requirements of care then he/she may be deemed to be negligent. Negligence could involve failing to elicit information relevant to the call or presenting complaint or giving wrong advice. It is sensible, therefore, for nurses to have indemnity insurance to protect against a claim of negligence.

Although it is possible for a patient to sue a nurse for negligence, it is unusual; pursuing a claim against the employer under the principle of vicarious liability is more likely. In the case of a co-operative, there are established lines of accountability. GP principals are responsible for all the acts and omissions of any person employed by or acting on their behalf or that of their deputies. The GP with whom the patient is registered is responsible for all the acts and omission of the co-operative employees (including nurses). The exception appears to be when the employees, in this case nurses, are employed by an NHS trust but based in a GP co-operative. In this situation, the trust retains responsibility for the nurses in terms of vicarious liability.

The employing organisation may be called upon to demonstrate that it has given sufficient attention to the training, supervision and professional development of its staff. A range of indicators can be used as indirect measures of the quality of call management and many aspects of the call process should be audited routinely. Examples are the variation in call management patterns between nurses; evidence of unusually long calls which might indicate failure to refer the caller to a more appropriate agency; the completeness of call documentation; and evidence from taped records of the consistent use of 'safety talk' (the caller advised to call back if concerned or if the patient's condition deteriorates). Decision support software can automatically generate a range of reports which can be used to support ongoing professional development and training.

Other indicators of quality include the incidence of adverse health events and caller experience of the service. Constructive use of complaint data can similarly identify aspects of the service which need improvement. Patient satisfaction surveys can also be used to elicit information about the acceptability and outcome of telephone advice. It may also be possible to systematically follow up a sample of calls to see how many patients have subsequent GP contact, are admitted to hospital or die unexpectedly. Linking these data with indepth call content review can be used to identify any evidence of suboptimal assessment and advice giving. However, this kind of study involves an investment of resources that may be beyond many services; it also requires appropriate permission for access to medical records.

Guidelines and decision support

Training, decision support and audit are essential components of a safe, high-quality service. In terms of the UKCC *Scope of Professional Practice*[12] the nurse must ensure that they have adequate educational preparation and competence to undertake any aspect of their role but particularly those that would fall outside the traditional remit. A recent enquiry in Ayrshire, Scotland, into care provided by a co-operative employing nurses highlighted the importance of adequate education and support, though the co-operative was exonerated in the cases studied.

Texts which provide guidelines for telephone consultation in general practice[13] are a useful resource for training and information and some co-operatives have produced their own guidelines and protocols for nurse telephone consultation. However, given the complex and varied nature of primary care problems, the value of these may be limited during consultations because of the time it takes to search for information manually.

Computerised decision support

Computerised decision support systems can be used contemporaneously to provide decision support and also document the consultation. There are two main types of decision support software available: those driven by protocol and algorithm and those designed to use guidelines. A protocol-driven or algorithmic approach provides a structured pathway of questions and answers which systematically prioritises the urgency of the patient's needs and identifies the appropriate level of advice that should be given. The strength of this approach is that it is likely to minimise risk. However, its disadvantage is that it may overwhelm the patient with closed questioning at the expense of discovering their underlying concerns and expectations. It may lead to longer call lengths and may tend to err excessively towards caution. At least two algorithm-based systems developed in the USA are now available in the UK. Evaluation of the safety and efficacy of such systems within the NHS is needed.

The second approach, a guideline-based system, is likely to encourage greater flexibility and judgement from the individual nurse by providing a structure for the consultation. It provides a series of prompts for assessment and suggested levels of response based on symptom complexes. However, it may be less safe in the hands of inadequately trained staff. The TAS used by WILCODOC and HARMONI utilises this approach. TAS was designed in the UK and is intended to encourage a greater search for symptoms before making a judgement about urgency and healthcare requirements. It was developed with an expert panel to model and embody within the software the processes used by clinicians in telephone assessment and decision making. By the end of 1998, it was being used by over 30 out-of-hours organisations in the UK.

The future of nurse telephone consultation in 24-hour primary care

Nurse telephone consultation is rapidly becoming an accepted approach to providing patient care and its profile is high in the UK. Its emergence within out-of-hours primary care has modified the care pathways traditionally available to patients. Specifically, nurse telephone consultation intervenes at the point of access to primary care and many patients therefore now have their out-of-hours needs managed entirely by a nurse. It seems likely that employment of nurses to assess and offer advice to out-of-hours callers will accelerate as the evidence supporting the safety and efficacy of this approach grows. However, the importance of training, organisational development and ongoing audit and quality improvement needs to be stressed if the quality of services is to be assured. These issues are discussed further in Chapter Eleven. We also need to know more about the health outcomes for callers who accept telephone advice, especially as poor care decisions may not always culminate in measurable adverse events. This is likely to be a high priority for further research.

NHS Direct

In parallel with nurses' growing involvement in out-of-hours care, NHS Direct, the new health telephone line for the NHS, is being implemented. This will give access to nurse telephone consultations throughout the day and night, with the whole of England to be covered by the end of 2000. Originally conceived as a service to manage the demand for emergency care in the community, the scope of NHS Direct will be much broader and ultimately it may become the main gateway to the NHS, providing 'easier and faster advice and information for people about health, illness and the NHS so that they are better able to care for themselves and their families'.[14]

But how will NHS Direct interface with primary care? The objectives of NHS Direct and the speed of its planned implementation seem likely to affect the provision of out-of-hours primary care. There were expectations that many people calling NHS Direct would be seeking health information rather than medical advice, but early evidence from NHS Direct pilot sites suggests that the proportion of symptom-related calls is very high. At this stage when most of the country is yet to be covered by the service, there has been little opportunity for NHS Direct to explain to the public the scope of its service, but if the proportion of medical advice calls to NHS Direct remains high, integration with primary care will be critically important to ensure that seamless care is delivered and duplication is avoided. Although as yet there are few data on the calls to NHS Direct, if the reasons for calling are consistent with current A&E and out-of-hours demand it is likely that the majority of calls will be of a primary care nature. The location of NHS Direct call centres may have an impact on how calls are handled and the extent to which this is integrated into existing service provision. The Department of Health has emphasised the need for integration with primary care and with this in mind, the potential strengths and limitations of basing NHS Direct within ambulance services, GP co-operatives or A&E departments are set out in Table 7.1.

NHS Direct is envisaged to be a largely nurse-delivered service, with approximately 1000 whole-time-equivalent nurse posts required[15] at a time when nurse recruitment and retention difficulties in the NHS are frequently reported. Early feedback from NHS Direct pilot sites suggests that NHS Direct is attracting nurses back into practice. There may be scope for other health personnel, paramedics for example, to perform a telephone triage role and at least one such study is already in progress. Any such developments, though, should be the subject of rigorous studies to explore their safety and efficacy before being adopted widely.

Table 7.1:   Potential strengths and limitations of three call centre locations for the delivery of NHS Direct

	Strengths	Limitations
Ambulance services	• Existing robust communications technology • Long-standing experience of call centre management • Longer term potential to manage category 'C' 999 calls through NHS Direct (subject to change in legislation) • Already serve large populations	• Integration with primary care has to be negotiated, from what to do for callers who need urgent GP care to providing medical cover for the service • Callers referred to GP co-operatives may be re-triaged • Limited experience of employing nurses • Command and control culture at odds with the philosophy of NHS Direct • Limited understanding of the primary care-type nature of calls to NHS Direct
GP co-operative	• Already provide out-of-hours call management to the public • Fully integrated with primary care • Critical mass of experienced nurse advisers may already be in place	• Call centre infrastructure less well developed than in ambulance services • Service currently provided for registered patients rather than for a geographical population • Few co-operatives have the organisational infrastructure to provide a 24-hour service for populations of 1.5–2 million people
Accident and emergency department	• Already manages telephone calls from the public and have triage systems in place • Facilitates inviting callers to attend A&E when clinically necessary • Potential to redirect primary care workload away from A&E	• Establishment of separate accommodation with dedicated personnel has to be specified • Tendency to invite callers to attend A&E • Difficult to balance role of telephone adviser with the other demands in a busy unit

References

1   OFTEL (1998) *Annual Report*. OFTEL, London.

2   Crouch R, Dale J (1998) Telephone triage – how good are the decisions ? (Part 2). *Nursing Standard*. **12**(35): 33–9.

3   Dale J, Crouch R (1997) It's good to talk. *Health Service J*. **107**(5536): 24–6.

4   Ott JE, Bellaire J, Machotka P, Moon JB (1974) Patient management by telephone by child health associates and pediatric house officers. *J Med Educ*. **49**: 596–600.

5   Bradley Brown S (1974) Use of the telephone by pediatric house staff: a technique for pediatric care not taught. *J Pediatr*. **84**(1): 117–19.

6   Greitzer L, Stapleton B, Wright L, Wedgewood RJ (1976) Telephone assessment of illness by practising pediatricians. *J Pediatr*. **88**(5): 880–2.

7   Perrin EC, Goodman HC (1978) Telephone management of acute paediatric illnesses. *NEJM*. **298**(3): 130–5.

8   Evans RJ, McCabe M, Allen H, Rainer T, Richmond PW (1993) Telephone advice in the accident and emergency department: a survey of current practice. *Arch Emerg Med*. **10**: 216–19.

9   Lattimer V, George S, Thompson F *et al.* (1998) Safety and effectiveness of nurse telephone consultation in out of hours primary care: randomised controlled trial. *BMJ*. **317**: 1054–9.

10   Crouch R, Patel A, Williams S, Dale J (1996) An analysis of telephone calls to an inner-city accident and emergency department. *J R Soc Med*. **89**: 324–8.

11   Dale J, Crouch R, Lloyd D (1998) Primary care: nurse-led telephone triage and advice out of hours. *Nursing Standard*. **12**(47): 41–5.

12   United Kingdom Central Council for Nursing, Midwifery and Health Visiting (1994) *The Scope of Professional Practice*. UKCC, London.

13   Jessop J, Armstrong E, Foster J, Aukland R (1998) *Conducting Telephone Consultations: a two day experiential course for GPs. Facilitators Pack*. Lambeth, Southwark and Lewisham Out of Hours Project. King's College School of Medicine and Dentistry, London.

14   Department of Health (1998) *The New NHS*. HMSO, London.

15   College of Health (1998) *Developing NHS Direct*. College of Health, London.

CHAPTER EIGHT

Nurse-led minor injury units

Emma Jefferys and Alistair Stinson

Introduction

Hospital accident and emergency (A&E) services are under increasing pressure due to the steady rise in demand;[1] 14 million people attended A&E departments in England alone during 1996–97.[2] It has been estimated that a substantial proportion of patients who attend A&E departments could be treated more appropriately elsewhere: at home; within primary care; or by new models of care developed for those patients who require urgent treatment but not specialist hospital care.[3]

New models of care have developed in many parts of the country for patients with minor injuries. Such patients have traditionally gained access to care at an A&E department or at their GP surgery or have treated themselves. In the last ten years, a number of reports and policy documents have looked at services for these patients. In 1988, the Royal College of Surgeons issued a working party report,[4] which the NHS Executive followed in 1994 with a descriptive study of services providing care for patients with minor injuries.[5] This study concluded that there was significant potential for cost savings in services and for improvements in efficiency. In the same year, a literature review was published by the University of Sheffield[6] and in 1996 the Audit Commission's report on A&E services included a review of minor injury services.[7]

These have been joined by many individual service evaluations, most of which have not been published or disseminated.[8–13] Other recent research includes an economic evaluation of the range of service models used to provide care for patients with minor injuries undertaken by the London Health Economics Consortium as part of the NHS Executive Health Technology Assessment Programme.[14]

The number and variety of minor injury services have expanded rapidly, with 293 individual services now identified as operational across the UK. Many are delivered solely by nurses, although almost all obtain telephone advice or other support, when required, either from medical staff in neighbouring A&E departments or local GPs. Some services have established links with out-of-hours services, either where nursing staff are involved in offering telephone assessment and advice or where premises are shared with out-of-hours organisations. Sometimes on-call support is provided by telemedical link to an A&E department.

This chapter will describe some of the service models currently available in the UK for the treatment of patients with minor injuries and offer a classification system for this wide range of services. This will be followed by a discussion of their key features, with particular attention to the interface issues with out-of-hours primary care. Finally, important issues to consider when planning a service will be outlined, together with possible future directions for these services.

Definition

There is no standard definition of a minor injury service. It is usually considered to be a local service for those suffering from a complaint which is not serious enough to require treatment or investigation at a fully equipped A&E department, but too serious to be treated at home. Care offered by a minor injury service differs from that provided within conventional primary care in that the aim is limited to providing acute episodic care for a predefined range of minor injuries.

In their 1994 study, the NHS Executive used a three-part definition for minor injury units:

- an open access, self-referral minor injury and ailments service for ambulatory patients that may also see patients referred by GPs
- a service more akin to that provided by an A&E department than by GPs in their surgeries, but which will overlap the work of both A&E and GPs
- a service for the treatment of minor injuries which do not fulfil the continuing care role of GPs and do not require inpatient facilities.

It is generally recognised that due to their wide diversity, any individual minor injury unit can only be defined by the services on offer, the scope of which reflect many factors, including:

- facilities available and access to on-site services such as X-ray and pharmacy
- age and location of the service and characteristics of the catchment population

- nature, qualifications and experience of the staff providing the service
- scope and scale of medical support to the unit
- links with local A&E departments and primary care
- access to specialist opinion and referral
- opening hours
- the use of nurse practitioner protocols (such as for issuing drugs and radiology requests)
- whether or not ambulance-borne cases are accepted.

Although many minor injury services are located on the site of an old A&E department or community hospital casualty department, a number coexist with other emergency services (sit within A&E departments or primary healthcare facilities), and an increasing number have developed as entirely new services. Box 8.1 gives a simple classification of minor injury services based on some aspects of the location and organisational model adopted by a particular service. Table 8.1 sets out some of the advantages and disadvantages that tend to be associated with each model.

Box 8.1: Types of minor injury service that are provided according to organisational model

Stand-alone unit
Care is delivered by highly trained and experienced nurses. Nurses often also lead the service, with back-up medical cover often provided by A&E medical staff or GPs either directly or via a telemedical link.

Within primary care centre or general practice
The service is usually GP led, nurse delivered and often linked to out-of-hours care. Telephone consultations and triage are often included.

In a hospital without an A&E department
Care is provided either by dedicated nurses or ward nurses, with on-call support provided by local GPs or A&E medical staff either directly or via a telemedical link.

Based within an existing A&E department
Patients with minor complaints triaged with other A&E patients, but may wait in a separate queue and be treated in a separate area. The service is usually delivered by either nurses or junior doctors.

Table 8.1: Advantages and disadvantages associated with different models of minor injury services

	Type of Unit			
	Stand-alone unit	Within primary care	In hospital that lacks an A&E	Part of A&E department
Advantages for A&E services	Can reduce pressure on local A&E department.	Can reduce pressure on local A&E and may help avoid hospital admission.	Can reduce pressure on local A&E and other departments if back-up clinics available on site.	Allows appropriate mix of staff to deal with minor injuries and may help reduce waits for more serious cases.
Advantages for local people	Provides local, accessible service, which may be more appropriate than A&E or GP.	Provides integrated local emergency and primary care service, with wider scope of service.	Provides local service, usually with shorter waits than A&E, and with good access to diagnostic and referral facilities.	Avoids confusion about which service to use, as only one point of entry. One-stop care can be assured for almost all injury-related problems.
Advantages for primary care	Local service which can reduce pressure on GPs. May be opportunity for out-of-hours links or telephone triage.	May help ensure appropriate care provided in the most appropriate environment and potential for links to support other areas of primary care service (i.e. out-of-hours service or practice nurse). Can reduce pressure on GPs.	Provides local emergency service, accessible for patients, integrated with diagnostic and referral services, but without the pressure of A&E. Potential for out-of-hours links or combined telephone triage.	Improved A&E service for patients with both minor and major injuries. Best possible access to back-up and other facilities. May also reduce pressure on GPs.

Table 8.1: Continued

	Type of Unit			
	Stand-alone unit	**Within primary care**	**In hospital that lacks an A&E**	**Part of A&E department**
Advantages for nurses	Extension of role, development of autonomous practice and links created to other local services.	Clinical support for nurses available, so extension of role possible, with potential for wider scope of service.	Extension of role, ability to refer to back-up facilities, and with potential for extra training from on-site staff.	Extension of role, with good on-site support and extra training. Can also keep up to date with A&E skills.
Disadvantages	Small services may not be cost effective, due to low activity levels, limited scope of service or lack of back-up facilities, protocols or support. Staff in such small units can become deskilled. May duplicate other local service provision.	Diagnostic support to the service may be limited and nurses may in actual fact have a reduced role if the service is GP led. May also duplicate services provided elsewhere in the locality and dual role of service may confuse patients.	Small services may not be cost effective, due to low activity levels or limited scope of service, especially if limited access to back-up facilities. Possibility for lack of integration with primary care and clinical isolation. May need to advertise scope of service on offer to ensure demand is appropriate.	Tendency for staff dedicated to minor injury service to be pulled into the major side of the A&E service when there are staff shortages. Harder to maintain links with primary care. Potential problems if patients with minor injuries are seen to wait for shorter periods than some others.

Key features

All minor injury services sit at the interface between the primary, community and secondary care sectors. Depending on the type of service model implemented, the service may be closer in terms of organisation, location, staffing or case mix to one or other of the different sectors. Key features of minor injury services are described below, with particular attention given to how these differ between services and the extent to which different factors encourage the success of particular arrangements.

Location

The expansion in the numbers of minor injury services has been experienced across the whole range of service sectors and geographical locations (including rural, inner city, suburban, market town). These different conditions have resulted in a variety of service types. The largest increases in new services have been within the primary and secondary care sectors (38% of services that responded to a questionnaire in the primary care sector had opened since 1995, as had 53% of services in the secondary care sector).[14] This is mainly because these types of services are a recent development within primary care and in secondary care, many minor injury services have been developed as the result of emergency services reconfigurations. Minor injury services within the community care sector have tended not to be new services but the refocusing of existing minor casualty departments.

The type of service sector in which the minor injury service is located has implications for the extent to which back-up facilities are available on site. This includes the level of clinical expertise and the availability of review clinics and outpatient departments that can be referred to at the site. In addition, the availability of facilities such as on-site X-ray and pharmacy results in many more episodes of care which can be completed at the unit, without the need for patients to be transferred or referred to another site or service. Respondents to the 1998 national survey of minor injury services reported that 62% had immediate access to X-ray (35% of these with access at all times) and 43% had immediate access to pharmacy (47% of these with access at all times the service operates).[14]

Figure 8.1 gives the profile of types of condition presented to a typical minor injury service.[14] Broken down by sector, considerably fewer primary care-based minor injury services treated fractures (55%) than those in either the community or secondary care sectors and only 80% treated head injuries. The scope of practice is strongly correlated with access to X-ray facilities in all sectors.

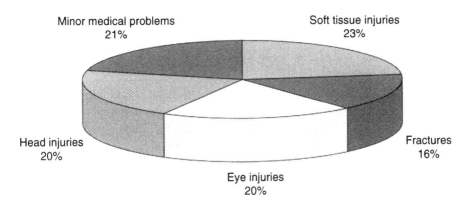

Figure 8.1:   Case mix presented to a typical minor injury service

Geographical location has a major impact on the type and scope of minor injury services. For example, in rural areas primary care-based services are more likely, while district general hospital-based services are more likely to serve suburban and inner-city populations; community hospital-based services mainly serve market towns and mixed suburban areas. Services in more rural locations are less likely to have nearby A&E departments to whom patients can be referred. This can result either in more restrictive protocols, ensuring patients do not attend the unit if there is any possibility that they will need to be transferred to an A&E, or more inclusive protocols because of the lack of alternative service provision.

In fact, rural services that are more distant from A&E departments have been found to be much more likely to accept ambulance-borne cases (89% of rural services compared to 29% of those in inner cities).[14] This finding clearly has implications for the clinical safety of units, as well as the staffing of ambulance services and personnel training requirements.

Easy access to services by patients (particularly in terms of time and cost) is a concern for all units and any new service has to be considered in relation to the other services provided in the locality. This is vital when attempting to maximise the use of limited healthcare resources and in particular to avoid duplication of services. Similarly, ensuring a safe, viable, effective and appropriately used service requires the development of good links with neighbouring A&E departments and local primary care.

As minor injury units tend to be located near to their catchment populations, the opportunities for collaboration with primary care services should be considerable. The involvement of GPs and other primary healthcare professionals with minor injury services has ranged from helping to develop assessment and treatment protocols, providing medical support to the unit, to providing first-line care in some stand-alone and community-based sites.

There are also a number of opportunities for joint working in the area of out-of-hours care, building on some of the recent developments such as telephone triage by nurses, telephone consultations for patients and provision of a central base (see below).

Two-thirds of minor injury services are open for 24 hours a day either during the week, at the weekend or both.[14] However, many of the individual service evaluations conducted have reported that very small numbers of patients attended the services between the hours of 11.30 pm and 8.30 am approximately, raising concerns over cost effectiveness at these times. In addition, there are sometimes fears for the physical safety of staff at small isolated units at night.

Clearly, there is a need to ensure that local people have access to an appropriate emergency service but the aim should be to avoid duplication of services. Efforts should be made to ensure that in areas where an out-of-hours service and a minor injury service are operating at night, there is a single telephone number and central call centre, enabling all patients to be triaged against the same protocols to the most appropriate service. In addition, sharing premises should lead to more efficient use of resources and improved staff safety and the costs to each service should be reduced dramatically. It will enable the best use of the skills of the staff available for both services. These possibilities should also be considered for the weekend period; only 8% of minor injury services reported that they were closed at weekends.[14]

Some services have already moved in this direction, for example at Swanage Hospital in Dorset and at Tamworth Hospital in Staffordshire. At both hospitals there are joint telephone answering/advice services for patients contacting the minor injury unit or phoning their GP out of hours. These are staffed by experienced minor injury unit nurses. Both services have found that nurses using computerised decision support can manage around 50% of out-of-hours calls with advice alone. This provides many benefits. Not only does it relieve the GPs of much of their out-of-hours workload, but it makes more efficient use of the minor injury unit's staff, particularly during night-time hours when their workload may otherwise be very limited. It also helps to raise the profile of the minor injury unit within the local community. This helps ensure that patients receive a smooth, high-quality service whilst avoiding duplication. It also gives greater development of the nurses' role and so may improve their job satisfaction. From the evaluations of these services, it appears that patients are highly satisfied and like the contact with a nurse and GPs perceive the service as providing efficient and effective care. The nurses can arrange to see the patient at the unit if a face-to-face consultation is required before referring the patient, if necessary, to a GP.

Protocols

Protocols are an essential part of any nurse-led minor injury service. They are likely to be most effective when developed in partnership with local clinicians (such as radiologists, pharmacists, GPs and other primary care professionals). They should define the scope of service at that unit and are dependent on a number of factors, including the level of clinical back-up, facilities, staff confidence, training and expertise. It is also important to define the overall aim of the service; for instance, whether it is to treat minor to moderate injuries (that is, closer to that of an A&E department) or be capable of treating minor illnesses as well as minor injuries (that is, more akin to that provided within primary care).

Protocols should help to ensure consistency in the management of particular problems, identify a framework for audit and encourage collaboration and clear lines of communication between nurses and other members of the healthcare team. Clearly, if their value is to be sustained, they must be dynamic and constantly revisited, reviewed and updated. Major barriers to services have been encountered where basic requirements are excluded from protocols, for example nurses ordering X-rays (where this service is available) and administering certain pharmaceuticals for certain conditions against clearly defined protocols.

The appropriateness of treating minor illness and other problems traditionally seen by a GP or referred to the practice nurse within services set up predominantly to provide care for patients with minor injuries is a hotly debated point. It has been argued that the health service is 'paying for the same service twice' but the marginal cost of treating these cases will usually be limited to minor items such as dressings and removing them is unlikely to change the staff profile.

Staffing

The skill mix and grade of staff employed influences the scope of practice that is possible. Nursing staff providing minor injury services often have a wide range of skills that can range from GP practice nurses, to nurses with experience of working in A&E departments, to highly trained emergency nurse practitioners. Clearly, different skills and experiences will be required in different service settings. However, the most advanced protocols can only be adopted in situations where the service is provided by highly trained and experienced staff, who have adequate support both within and outside the service.

The variety in the nature of staff providing minor injury services is partly due to the lack of national guidelines on the skill mix necessary for this type of service and the limit on nationally approved emergency nurse practitioner courses. The ENB A33 (Developing Autonomous Practice) is currently offered by five universities and although there are other nurse practitioner courses available, there are no national guidelines from professional bodies indicating what courses should cover or what the expected level of achievement should be.

One emergency nurse practitioner training course, provided by Thames Valley University and Central Middlesex Hospital NHS Trust, requires 120 hours of student contact time, 120 hours of student-directed study and 80 hours of student clinical placement over 24 weeks. The course covers a broad set of issues (Box 8.2). It is aimed at nurses working in an advanced minor injury service based in a hospital without an A&E department, but linked to the main A&E department. The aim is to train staff to deal with the types of case outlined in Box 8.3.

Box 8.2:   Emergency nurse practitioner syllabus

- Ethical and legal issues
- Systematic patient assessment
- Anatomy and physiology of upper and lower limbs
- Orthopaedic minor injuries
- Ophthalmic injuries
- Ear, nose and throat problems

- Paediatric minor injuries/ailments
- Elderly patients
- Psychology of ageing
- Sociology of ageing
- Psychiatric patients
- Ethnic, cultural and social issues

Box 8.3:   Types of case that minor injury nurses should be capable of managing

- Lacerations with no underlying damage
- Superficial puncture wounds
- Abrasions and bruises
- Sprains and strains
- Minor surgical, e.g. removal of foreign bodies, trephining subungual haematoma
- Fractures
- Minor eye conditions
- Minor head injury
- Dressings

- Toothache to include analgesia
- Stings and bites
- Superficial burns to <2–5% of body surface
- Minor allergic reactions
- Removal of ear and nose studs; rings; contact lenses; tampons
- Plaster of Paris problems
- Uncomplicated nasal bone fracture
- Epistaxis including nasal packing
- Minor medical conditions

It is now widely recognised that well-trained nurse practitioners can offer a high-quality service. Nurse practitioners have often been reported to have a more holistic approach to patient care than doctors in the same situation and have been shown (where properly trained) to request and interpret correctly a limited range of X-rays to at least the same standard as senior house officers.[15] High-quality minor injury services tend to have few problems with recruiting and retaining nursing staff, particularly where opportunities are given for staff to receive extra training. Nurses' workloads cannot be increased without adequate support, training and resources.

Issues to consider when planning a service

Evidence is lacking about whether one type of minor injury service is more cost effective or more efficient or of higher quality than another. The optimal type of service will depend on the local circumstances. Whatever the type of service, there are a number of important markers of success that can be used when evaluating an existing service or planning a new service (Box 8.4).

Box 8.4: Factors associated with the effectiveness of minor injury services

Success criteria
- Good links with local A&E departments and primary care services
- Complementary to local emergency services
- Good links to local outpatient services
- Receive referrals from local GPs
- Low transfer rate to local A&E department
- Nurses able to dispense against protocol
- Strong clinical and managerial support
- Ongoing training and development of skills

Unhealthy signs
- Limited or no links with local A&E departments and primary care services
- Duplication of other emergency services
- Lack of ownership by staff in unit
- Service not defined by staff as separate
- Low activity levels
- Restrictive protocols
- Managerial and clinical isolation
- Poorly identified location and poor access

Where these services are available:
- Ability of nurses to X-ray or refer for X-ray
- Nurses able to refer to outpatient and review clinics
- Good integration with on-site services

Where these services are available:
- Medical approval required to order X-rays
- Lack of interest from A&E consultant
- Service interrupted by pressure of main A&E

In addition, the following checklist will help to ensure a high-quality, cost-effective service.

- Develop evidence-based, regularly updated protocols in conjunction with local experts, based on skills and experience of staff and distance from nearest A&E.
- Develop good working relationships with local A&E departments and primary care and open dialogue with other emergency services about sharing of facilities, staff and costs.
- Good access to diagnostic facilities, pharmacy and specialist clinics and appropriate referral routes established to alternative services when necessary.
- Appropriate skill mix between triage staff, treatment staff and clerical staff.
- High-level managerial support and commitment.
- Ensure training opportunities are maximised and regular clinical audits carried out.
- Opening times optimal for the needs of the population being served.
- Clear, multipronged advertising material, aimed at all sectors of the community, taking account of the characteristics of the local area (ethnicity, elderly population, etc.).
- Ensure adequate external signposting in the locality of the unit.

Future of minor injury services

Minor injury services delivered predominantly by nurses require a strong supportive relationship with medical colleagues in order to be able to offer a wide range of services and carry out formalised referral procedures. Even so, the ultimate aim of nurse-led minor injury services should not be to respond to medical overload but to make the maximum use of what nursing can offer, ensuring cost-effective services are maintained across the board.

There are particular opportunities for the minor injury services and out-of-hours services in a locality to develop closer working relationships, particularly as most minor injury services are open at weekends and many open overnight, with highly trained staff available to treat patients. Ideally, both services should be located on the same site, even if the minor injury service does not operate at night. Combining the main premises of a GP co-operative with a minor injury service can promote cost-effective, high-quality, seamless care. This can include a shared central telephone call centre to aid access to information and advice for the public and to ensure that patients are receiving consistent triage advice.

However, as with all new and rapidly changing services, there are a number of outstanding issues both about the interface between minor injuries and out-of-hours services and about minor injury services more generally. These include the following.

- How will minor injury services and out-of-hours services work jointly to gain the most from NHS Direct?
- Should minor injury services based in primary care be integrated with GP practice nurse drop-in services?
- Is there a niche for nurse-led minor injury units whilst A&E departments continue to employ GPs in A&E to provide a primary care service?
- Will minor injury services on hospital sites without A&E departments become just another route into direct-access diagnostic and treatment services?
- How can nurse-led minor injury services provide adequate support for junior doctors in the assessment of patients?

References

1   Hallam L, Wilkin D, Roland M (1996) *24 Hour Responsive Healthcare.* University of Manchester, National Primary Care Research and Development Centre, Manchester.

2   Department of Health (1997) *Statistical Bulletin 1997/20.* HMSO, London.

3   Dale J, Dolan B (1996) Do patients use minor injury units appropriately? *J Public Health Med.* **18**(2): 152–6.

4   Royal College of Surgeons of England (1988) *Report of the Working Party on the Management of Patients with Minor Injuries.* Royal College of Surgeons of England, London.

5   NHS Management Executive (1994) *A Study of Minor Injury Services.* NHSME, Leeds.

6   Read S (1994) *Patients with Minor Injuries: a literature review of options for their treatment outside major A&E departments or occupational health settings.* Sheffield Centre for Health and Related Research, University of Sheffield.

7   Audit Commission (1996) *By Accident or Design – improving A&E services in England and Wales.* HMSO, London.

8   Bevan H, Morris-Thompson T (1993) *Care Must Not be a Casualty – a strategic review of minor casualty services in Leicestershire.* Leicestershire Health, Leicester.

9   Dale J (1993) *Health Care in Gravesend: what future for the minor casualty centre?* King's College School of Medicine and Dentistry, Department of General Practice and Primary Care, London.

10   Heaney DJ (1997) *Evaluation of the Minor Injuries Clinic at the Western General Hospital, Edinburgh. Final Report.* GP Research Group, University of Edinburgh.

11 London Health Economics Consortium (1997) *Minor Injuries at Mount Vernon and Watford General Hospitals.* Harrow, Hillingdon and West Hertfordshire Health Authorities, London.

12 Palmer C (1996) *Evaluation of Wembley Minor Accident and Treatment Service.* Central Middlesex NHS Hospital Trust, London.

13 Woodruffe C (1996) *St Albans Minor Injury Unit – a second evaluation.* Hertfordshire Health Authorities, Herts.

14 Haycock J, Jefferys E, Clark J, Ryder S (1998) *Economic evaluation of different service models for the management of minor injuries – phase 1 descriptive study.* Proceedings of the Third International Conference on Strategic Issues in Healthcare Management: Managing Quality and Controlling Cost, 2–4 April, St Andrews, Scotland.

15 Freij R (1996) Radiographic interpretation by nurse practitioners in a minor injuries unit. *J Accident Emerg Med.* **13**(1): 41–3.

CHAPTER NINE

Responding to patients with particular needs

Cathy Shipman and Jeremy Dale

Introduction

During the 1990s the rise in out-of-hours workload became the main impetus for implementing new service responses to relieve the pressure felt by GPs. The principal concern for GPs was to manage expressed patterns of demand more efficiently and effectively. In the planning and development of co-operatives and other new service arrangements, relatively little attention was given to the diversity of needs that occur within out-of-hours periods. As is the case when any change in service provision occurs, a development which may be beneficial to one group of patients may inadvertently compromise the access to appropriate levels of care for other groups of individuals. There is increasing evidence that the new forms of out-of-hours service delivery may be inadequate to meet the needs of particular groups of patients. These include those with long-term illness, such as the mentally ill or patients receiving palliative care, and those who have difficulty communicating over the phone, for example those with language or hearing difficulties.

Many of the issues relevant to the equity of service provision need to be addressed within the context of 24-hour service delivery. Help seeking and service use out of hours cannot be divorced from issues around equity and accessibility within hours. However, it is within the out-of-hours period, when the availability of health services is limited and other systems of support may be lacking, that inequalities within the health service may be revealed more starkly.

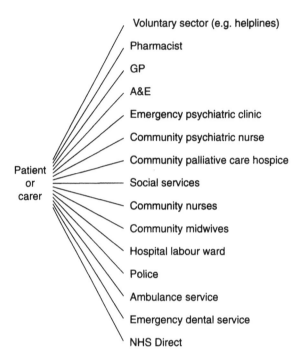

Figure 9.1: Sources of out-of-hours help for patients and carers (LSL Out of Hours Project report)

Success in gaining appropriate out-of-hours care depends on a number of factors: knowing what care is available, knowing how to access it and being able to do so. Figure 9.1 shows a range of out-of-hours service providers that generally are available across most health authority districts. Service providers frequently have little understanding of the nature or extent of each other's out-of-hours arrangements, nor how these can best be accessed. There is often a need for greater co-ordination and collaboration between services out of hours, as well as networking between statutory and non-statutory agencies.

In this chapter we consider some of the groups of people who experience particular difficulty in gaining the help they need out of hours. These include:

- those who may have an urgent need for community-based specialist help
- those who have difficulty gaining access to the healthcare system as a consequence of disability or disadvantage
- those who have difficulty in communicating needs.

In the second part of the chapter we present different examples of specialist provision and consider the implications these have for out-of-hours general medical services.

Needs and difficulties of certain groups

A needs assessment exercise undertaken in south London as part of a process of developing new systems of out-of-hours care raised many concerns about the accessibility and availability of care for certain members of the local population.[1] The four main issues that emerged, although specific to the metropolis, probably apply to most parts of the country.

Lack of availability of community-based specialist help

Many community-based specialist services that are available during normal working hours are lacking during out-of-hours periods. This reflects historical patterns of commissioning and the boundaries between different provider organisations. This may lead to needs not being met or being met inappropriately, particularly for those with mental health or palliative care needs.

Inappropriate responses

Palliative care and hospice services, for example, reported that on occasions patients were admitted to hospital when they could have been cared for at home if appropriate advice and support had been sought from them by the attending GP. This may reflect lack of knowledge and understanding of the services that are available or a lack of confidence or willingness of doctors to support palliative care in the community. Mental health groups also stated that limited social worker and community psychiatric nurse availability out of hours lead GPs to sometimes seek admission for patients suffering from mental health problems who could otherwise have been maintained in the community.

Difficulties in accessing help

Some groups, such as the homeless, refugees/asylum seekers or those away from home, were using A&E services because of non-registration with a local GP. Groups representing people suffering from physical, learning and mental disabilities and difficulties also reported problems in gaining access to services. Those who are blind or visually impaired may experience particular difficulty in attending an out-of-hours facility, as may people with physical disabilities.

Difficulties in communicating needs

For example, people with learning difficulties may have limited speech that may create difficulty in describing or interpreting the significance of particular symptoms. Carers reported difficulty in making contact with out-of-hours services and felt healthcare professionals often lacked appreciation of their problems. Language differences can provide an absolute barrier to service use out of hours and people with limited or no spoken English may have great difficulties in summoning help, for example in not being able to give a home address or respond to an answerphone message or receptionist.

Examples of groups requiring urgent community-based specialist help

Palliative care

Extent of need

On average 90% of the last year of life of patients with palliative care needs is spent at home, under the care of the primary healthcare team. Even when symptom management is effective, the progressive nature of terminal disease can lead to rapid unexpected deterioration in a patient's condition. Inevitably, this may occur during out-of-hours periods. An audit of a GP co-operative covering 210 000 patients in Cambridge identified 53 contacts for 40 terminally ill patients (2.4% of 2202 contacts during the month of August 1996).[2] A 'snapshot' of out-of-hours and emergency service use undertaken across Lambeth, Southwark and Lewisham over a four-day Easter weekend in 1996 found 1% of all contacts were made to a hospice, including planned care, but these contacts were only from patients registered with the hospice, whose geographical patch did not cover the entire district.[3]

Out-of-hours calls monitored to one specialist service over a three-month period identified the key areas of need for help to include new or worsening symptoms (for example pain, nausea and vomiting, restlessness and breathlessness), the anxiety of carers and/or the patient and the need for advice, for example on taking medication, or nursing care.[4]

Specialist support out of hours

Department of Health guidance (1995) recommends that patients and carers should be able to get 24-hour support from a healthcare professional who is aware of their circumstances, but the availability of out-of-hours specialist provision varies widely. Such support could be based in hospice, hospital or community nursing services.

In some areas 24-hour advice and support are available to terminally ill patients and their carers together with home visits as required, but in others telephone contact over limited hours only may be provided. A survey of 98 hospices in the UK and Ireland found only 60–70% of those with home care teams provided 24-hour and weekend cover.[5] While community night nursing services exist, they are becoming scarcer and more variable in provision. Marie Curie nurses provide 'hands-on' 24-hour nursing care in many areas, although the availability of such care can sometimes be inadequate to meet the needs of the last few weeks of a patient's life.

An example of a well-developed out-of-hours palliative care service is provided by St Christopher's Hospice in Sydenham, south London. This provides a community palliative care service that covers four health authority boundaries. It provides an out-of-hours telephone advice and on-call service to registered patients and their carers, as well as to healthcare professionals, each evening and night between 5.00 pm and 9.00 am and over weekends. A senior inpatient nurse receives the calls, filters out messages and information requests and passes the call on to the home care staff who either provide advice over the telephone or visit the patient if necessary. Dorothy House, Bradford-on-Avon, and Prospect Hospice, Swindon, provide similar examples of 24-hour provision of specialist advice to patients, carers and healthcare professionals that is available out of hours through inpatient staff.

Little evaluation of specialist out-of-hours palliative care has been undertaken in the UK. However, there is encouraging evidence from other countries. For example, the Motala hospital-based palliative home care programme in Sweden[6] enabled 89% of patients to die at home, partly through providing 24-hour availability of a doctor or nurse within 30 minutes. The study concluded that the immediate availability of professional help enabled patients and carers to face more problems at home, especially at night.

Primary care issues

Continuity of care is a key issue for patients with palliative care needs. A survey of deputising doctors undertaken in 1995 found that almost a third of GPs considered offering their home telephone number to patients who were in the last weeks of life.[7] A recent survey indicates that despite changes in out-of-hours arrangements, almost a quarter of GPs still claim to usually provide palliative care to their own patients, although this was more common amongst those using practice-based on-call arrangements.[8]

Avoidable hospital admissions may occur where GPs do not have access to medical notes and are unsure about care plans. Until recently, few GP co-operatives had developed specific policies for responding to the needs of palliative care patients. A national survey found that none had protocols concerning palliative care[9] and an audit of a Cambridge co-operative found that no information concerning patients making contact had been passed by GPs during the month of August 1996.[2] Little communication within the co-operative had occurred concerning second calls for help.

At a workshop held in November 1998 for the Macmillan Cancer Relief Programme of GP Facilitators in Cancer and Palliative Care, information was presented concerning a number of co-operatives where protocols and procedures are being developed to ensure adequate handover of information on patients who are terminally ill; effective availability of information within the co-operative; easy access to a range of palliative care drugs; and audits to ensure that quality of service provision is being maintained and improved.

The limited availability of district nursing night cover in many areas may lead to increased GP contacts and avoidable acute or hospice admissions. In Bradford, an out-of-hours district nursing service was developed in 1996 which amalgamated the evening, night and weekend service, developing specific referral criteria which included palliative care patients. Although yet to be fully evaluated, it is felt that the extension of district nursing care out of hours has successfully prevented acute hospital or hospice admissions.[10]

Greater interagency collaboration is likely to be necessary to ensure that GPs working out of hours have better access to specialist advice and support, whether working for co-operatives, deputising services or within practice-based arrangements. Patient-held records provide one means of enabling improved communication between within-hours and out-of-hours services and so may improve continuity of care. However, to be effective all visiting health and social care professionals need to make use of them.

Mental health needs

Extent of need

A questionnaire survey of 92 practices in East Riding Health District found that almost half of GP respondents had been called out more than five times in the previous two years to a patient with a mental health crisis and that three-quarters of these calls occurred out of hours.[11] While 75% of GP respondents said that they had contacted a psychiatrist and half a community nurse, concerns were voiced about the lack of availability of crisis help, delays in response and difficulties found in contacting services, particularly during out-of-hours periods.

An analysis of contacts with services over the Easter weekend in Lambeth, Southwark and Lewisham found that only 1% were to mental health services, the majority of which were unplanned contacts, 44% attending a clinic, 37% receiving telephone advice and 28% being visited at home.[3] When presenting complaints were considered across all service providers, the most frequently used services for those experiencing mental health problems were A&E departments, mental health services and GPs. For those who were suicidal, attempting deliberate self-harm or overdose, A&E departments and the ambulance service were the main points of contact.

Few community mental health services provide emergency out-of-hours care and both providers and user groups (MIND and National Schizophrenia Fellowship) have criticised the lack of specialist help that is available out of hours.[12] Even where services do exist, such as helplines, walk-in clinics and crisis teams, communication difficulties are frequently cited between different agencies, for example between GPs, the police and mental health and social service professionals, and confusion over appropriate roles, indicating the need for better co-ordination.[1]

A lack of 24-hour specialist psychiatric emergency services has led to urgent assessments and treatment being undertaken to an increasing extent in A&E departments and psychiatric hospital wards.[12] Patients with severe acute mental health problems, such as those who are psychotic, intoxicated from alcohol and drug ingestion or parasuicidal, present more frequently in most areas to A&E departments than to general practice. However, A&E departments are not the most appropriate environment for such patients because of their lack of space and privacy, bright lights and general lack of calm.

Specialist support

In most areas there is a clear need for greater 24-hour availability of key workers/community psychiatric nurses (CPN), mental health helplines, crisis counselling services and access to advice and assessment.[11] Some specialist services, however, do provide examples of good practice. In Birmingham, for instance, a 24-hour acute home treatment team was established in 1995 which included community mental health nurses, social workers, a psychologist and consultant psychiatrist cover. The team aimed to provide emergency psychiatric treatment at home for people with severe mental illness, following a referral through a psychiatrist. An evaluation has shown a reduction in unnecessary hospital admissions and a reduction in costs and users liked the 24-hour availability of help, even when this was purely telephone contact.[13] In Leeds an intensive home treatment team was developed which provided a 24-hour acute mental health service as an option to admission. The team have developed a comprehensive medication plan which includes medication prescribed by the GP and this plan is accessible to all health professionals involved as well as users.[14] The Maudsley Hospital in south-east London provides a 24-hour open access emergency clinic and the community division provides a home-visiting service between 5.00 pm and 9.00 am for GP referrals where urgent advice is required. A rapid-response out-of-hours service started in 1994 with three years funding from St Mary's Hospital and comprised a multidisciplinary team who visited the patient's home or GP's surgery. The largest group of GP referrals related to patients who were feeling suicidal. The service aimed to respond immediately to referrals for statutory assessment and managed admissions or arranged outpatient follow-up where appropriate. Other developments include CPN telephone support during the evening.

Telephone helplines provided by non-statutory services play an important role in responding to out-of-hours mental health crises (for example, the Samaritans and Saneline), though not all are available throughout the night.

Assessments for Sections 2 and 3 of the Mental Health Act require ideally a doctor who is a mental health specialist and a GP who knows the patient. As most GPs are now members of co-operatives or make use of deputising services, during out-of-hours periods there is little likelihood of patients seeing a GP familiar with their history or who has access to their records. A further accredited doctor (a specialist mental health consultant or senior registrar) is therefore usually called upon. Although this reduces the strain on out-of-hours GP services, it increases the demands being made on on-call psychiatrists. Developments in general practice out-of-hours care may well be creating additional difficulties for patients who require mental health assessments and for social workers when attempting to contact a GP who knows the patient.

Primary care issues

Lack of out-of-hours specialist mental health services to provide advice and for referral can create difficulties for GPs, as can the difficulty of contacting an emergency social worker who often has to cover a wide geographical patch out of hours. While in some areas there have been attempts to encourage close working between out-of-hours social services and general medical services, such as through both using the same base facilities, there are considerable organisational and historical factors that may militate against such developments.

A recent survey of GP co-operatives[9] indicated that some were developing or intending to develop protocols, policies or procedures concerning mental health problems and informal links with community psychiatric nurses and considering integration with mental health community teams. There is also potential to train more GPs to provide mental health assessments, but this appears to be more difficult to put into practice.

While relatively few out-of-hours contacts with GPs relate directly to mental illness, many reflect degrees of underlying anxiety, depression and other psychosocial problems which influence the extent to which patients cope and their thresholds for seeking care. A recent audit in south-east London found that participating GPs considered that about a third of calls had urgent psychological or emotional needs, often in the context of other physical problems.[15]

Difficulties in accessing services
The homeless

Extent of need

People who are homeless include those who are statutorily homeless and may be living in temporary accommodation, together with those sleeping on the streets. Many people who are homeless fail to register with a GP because of lack of a permanent address, high mobility and anticipation or experience of rejection. This is particularly so for the single homeless, for refugees and asylum seekers. Such individuals are therefore likely to have particular difficulty in accessing help out of hours.

The needs of homeless people are often complex and include poor health arising from cramped or outdoor living, poor diet and hygiene. Homeless people are likely to experience pressing psychological and social needs. The most common problems suffered include accidents and injuries, alcohol dependency, mental illness, drug dependence, respiratory disease and dermatological problems. A greater prevalence of tuberculosis, epilepsy and HIV infection has also been found and people sleeping on the streets are more prone to attack.

Many homeless people make use of A&E departments. This reflects lack of access to other primary care services, the prevalence of complex and urgent healthcare needs in this population and aspects of users' preference. A survey of people registering with 'no fixed abode' at an A&E department in south London found that over half (54%) attended outside working hours and over half of all homeless attenders said that they preferred coming to A&E despite 42% being aware of community medical facilities for the homeless.[16] However, a study by Shelter concluded that 57% of homeless attenders at University College Hospital, London, could have more 'appropriately' been seen by a GP.[17] There is a need to increase awareness and provision of accessible services for homeless people.

Specialist services

Specific out-of-hours services for the homeless are provided in some areas where the numbers of homeless are particularly great.[18] Examples in London include St Martins in the Field Social Care Unit which provides midweek and weekend services from an attached medical centre and Great Chapel Street Medical Centre in Westminster which provides primary care facilities during the day with access to the Kensington, Chelsea and Westminster GP co-operative during the evening. Homeless people in temporary accommodation – bed and breakfast or hostels – telephone the centre and are diverted to the GP co-operative, which then responds to their calls.

A 'rough sleepers' initiative has been developed in Leicester. This is a collaborative venture between a GP working in a night shelter and drop-in centre, housing advice and community care team representatives, hostel and shelter managers, outreach and resettlement officers, a psychologist and a psychiatric nurse.[19] The multidisciplinary team's aim is to improve clients' accommodation and almost half of the clients seen between January and July 1998 appeared to have benefited from the initiative. Interagency collaboration had enabled the team to understand much more about the remits and limitations of each other's work and so provide more mutual support to those working with the homeless.

A number of outreach teams (e.g. Crisis) provide multidisciplinary support at places where homeless people live, but the hours of availability are variable. A key feature of such outreach and fixed site facilities is to provide information on services available and they are a crucial link in the chain to enable homeless people to access both social support and health care out of hours.

Primary care issues

The difficulties faced by the homeless during out-of-hours periods reflect their lack of access to primary care services in general. A key aim, therefore, needs to be improvement in access to GPs' services within office hours. Some services have been developed to help the homeless gain access to primary care services. In Reading, for example, a specialist health visitor for the homeless was appointed in 1992, whose remit was to improve access to primary care services.[20] Although a within-hours appointment, she was able to restore contact between families visited and primary healthcare services, which then provided them with access to other forms of healthcare.

A further issue to consider is the accessibility of out-of-hours primary care centres run by co-operatives and deputising services. Like other disadvantaged groups, the homeless are unlikely to have the resources to travel far. Locating centres near A&E departments is likely to be advantageous, as the A&E is usually a well-known location served by public transport links.

Difficulties in communication

Language differences

Extent of need

It has been estimated that 23% of people from ethnic minority groups born in China, Bangladesh, India or Pakistan are unable to communicate effectively in English. Those with language and cultural differences may experience difficulty gaining access to primary care services in general and such difficulties are likely to be accentuated during the out-of-hours period. A survey of Chinese people working in 'takeaways' in Hull, for example, found that they were less likely than a white control group working in fish and chip shops to find surgery times convenient and, when needing urgent help, were more likely to request an ambulance or attend hospital in comparison to the 'white group' who tended to telephone their GP.[21]

Language differences are a barrier to service use out of hours, particularly when access to knowledgeable interpreters is limited. They can lead to a lack of knowledge about out-of-hours services available, arising from the inability to communicate effectively. A study undertaken with members of the Vietnamese community[22] demonstrated that very few of them were able to use GP out-of-hours services, largely because of the difficulty in communicating. A subsequent audit of the local GP co-operative revealed few people calling with limited spoken English, indicating that such residents do not attempt to use the service. In some cases, there is lack of awareness about the existence of out-of-hours GP services. Dialling 999 and waiting until the call was traced to their address was sometimes the only means known of gaining help other than by attending an A&E department. Children are often used as translators. The need for interpreters has been identified at A&E departments.[23]

Great difficulties can arise when attempting to summon help, for example through not being able to give a home address, respond to an answerphone message or telephonist or communicate needs to service providers. Particular difficulties may exist for those who lack family or friends to interpret and using children as interpreters can be particularly problematic for both the patient and the child. The elderly in particular are more likely to have less use of spoken English and potentially greater needs for accessible interpreting services.[24]

Needs will be greatest where the numbers of people from black and ethnic groups are highest, particularly within inner-city areas. For example, 26% of the population of Lambeth, Southwark and Lewisham are from black and ethnic groups representing a wide variety of cultural and language differences, including many refugees with little or no spoken English. While a range of interpreting services are provided across the three boroughs, residents can be unaware of these services or find them difficult to access during out-of-hours periods.

Specialist provision and primary care issues

Outreach community health services for black and ethnic groups tend not to provide out-of-hours cover. Frequently such provision is advice based and dependent on voluntary groups who tend to fluctuate according to funding available. During the day, some GPs fluent in specific languages are accessible to some ethnic groups, but out-of-hours GP co-operatives are seldom able to provide such availability in the wide range of languages that may be required. Interpreting services can enable access to primary care, but need to be widely known about and accessible to both patients and providers.

A study of Vietnamese refugees found considerable concern over lack of access to interpreters out of hours. Concerns were expressed about lack of access to health services when they or their children became ill and a 24-hour telephone interpreting service was felt to be needed.[25] The needs of those with no spoken English may remain hidden from providers of health-care service until mechanisms, such as interpreting services, are introduced to enable them to be expressed.

The way forward

In this chapter we have presented a range of complex needs which tend to be inadequately catered for by current out-of-hours arrangements. They illustrate the importance of considering out-of-hours needs, rather than just expressed levels of demand. Many issues have been highlighted concerning the equity and accessibility of services, the co-ordination of responses and achieving continuity of care. These need to be carefully thought about in the planning of out-of-hours services.

The examples of special needs discussed in this chapter are not meant to be comprehensive. Many other groups of people probably encounter similar difficulties although their exact form will vary from district to district and from individual to individual. Specific attention ought to be given to identifying unmet needs, as well as to responding efficiently to current levels of expressed demand. A variety of approaches may be required; these could include, for example, audits of practice populations or working with community group representatives and client populations. Working with local communities may help to disseminate information about available services, as well as providing a means of identifying the problems that individuals and groups are experiencing with current services.

Primary care groups draw together GP, community nursing, social service and lay perspectives and so provide a new context within which to identify and plan for the out-of-hours needs of groups with special difficulties. PCGs are in a strong position to influence the co-ordination and integration of out-of-hours services and they may encourage the development of innovative joint developments to meet out-of-hours healthcare needs more effectively.

Although GP out-of-hours services are frequently the first port of call, as illustrated here certain problems are likely to require more specialist knowledge or higher levels of support than co-operatives or deputising services are usually able to provide. However, for many special needs, appropriate out-of-hours help is limited and patchy. People who are receiving ongoing specialist care are more likely to have severe and complex out-of-hours problems and it appears that they often have difficulty in accessing appropriate out-of-hours services at times of acute need.

Improving accessibility

Many issues relating to the accessibility of out-of-hours services have been raised. GP co-operatives and deputising services need to consider how they can make their services more accessible to individuals who are disadvantaged or disabled. They should look at the entire pathway involved in decision making and accessing care, from how patients learn about the availability of their service, to the means of making telephone contact, to the care that is provided.

The availability and accessibility of interpreting services, for example, is important to consider and in all areas it should now be possible to address this using conference phoneline facilities. The siting of primary care centres is also important given the shift away from out-of-hours home visiting. The accessibility of centres should be considered, particularly for those with lack of resources to travel, as should the option of providing patient transport.

In many areas there is also a need to provide greater accessibility to 24-hour specialist advice and intervention if the needs of groups like the mentally ill or those requiring palliative care are to be adequately met. Without this, services such as A&E departments are often used and this may lead to inappropriate care.

However, issues affecting the accessibility of out-of-hours services cannot be addressed in isolation. They tend to reflect the difficulties that certain individuals and groups experience in accessing health services in general and so need to be addressed within a much broader context. For example, increasing the number of practices with whom the homeless are able to register would also help homeless people to access out-of-hours services.

Continuity of care

Achieving continuity of care across the interface between within-hours and out-of-hours care and across the interfaces between various care agencies is a key problem. Individuals with complex out-of-hours problems, such as those with palliative care or severe mental health needs, often find that they cannot contact a GP or other healthcare professional out of hours who is familiar with their history and current care requirements.

A range of actions may be helpful. These include taking a more strategic approach to co-ordinating care (see below), with the implementation of agreed protocols and guidelines. In the near future the greater use of IT across the health service should allow access to shared computer-held information at all times and this should have an important impact on promoting greater continuity of care. Clinical governance requirements (*see* Chapter Eleven) will also play a part and should lead to more explicit criteria being implemented and audited to ensure quality service provision out of hours for special needs groups.

Co-ordination of response

Access to appropriate levels of out-of-hours care for individuals and groups with special needs requires good working relationships between agencies, for example between GPs, A&E departments, mental health services and social services, as well as with non-statutory services. Explicit and accessible referral networks need to be developed and maintained. Achieving this requires dialogue between agencies and clarification of roles. It may also require staff training programmes and the implementation of referral and treatment protocols and guidelines. Information about the types of specialist service available locally, the care they provide and how this can be accessed should be disseminated and readily available to all professionals working out of hours and such data need to be frequently updated. Information technology may have an important part to play in supporting this process with the wider introduction of decision support systems. Issues relating to the co-ordination and integration of services are discussed further in Chapter Ten.

References

1   Dale J, Shipman C, Lacock L, Davies M (1996) Creating a shared vision of out of hours care: using rapid appraisal methods to create an interagency, community oriented, appropriate to service development. *BMJ*. **312**: 1206–10.

2   Barclay S, Rogers M, Todd C (1998) Communication between GPs and co-operatives is poor for terminally ill patients. *BMJ.* **315**: 1235–6.

3   Hollins L (1997) *A 'Snapshot' of Out of Hours and Emergency Services in Lambeth, Southwark and Lewisham Health Authority.* LSL Out of Hours Project, King's College School of Medicine and Dentistry, London.

4   Hatcliffe S, Smith P (1997) Open all hours. *Health Service J.* **107**: 40–1.

5   Johnson I, Rogers C, Biswas B, Ahmedzai S (1990) What do hospices do? A survey of hospices in the United Kingdom and Republic of Ireland. *BMJ.* **300**: 791–3.

6   Beck-Friis B, Strang P (1993) The organization of hospital-based home care for terminally ill cancer patients: the Motala model. *Palliat Med.* **7**: 93–100.

7   Boyd K (1995) The role of specialist home care teams: views of general practitioners in south London. *Palliat Med.* **9**: 138–44.

8   Shipman C, Addington-Hall J, Barclay S *et al.* (1999) Providing palliative care in primary care: are current 'out of hours' arrangements meeting with the satisfaction of GPs and district nurses? Paper submitted to the *Brit J Gen Pract.*

9   Payne F, Jessopp L, Dale J (1997) *Second National Survey of GP Co-operatives: a report.* LSL Out of Hours Project, King's College School of Medicine and Dentistry, London.

10 Sands G, Rayner S (1997) Night and day. *Health Service J.* **107**: 30–1.

11 Gray P, Baulcombe S (1996) Crisis de coeur. *Health Service J.* **106**: 24–5.

12 Johnson S, Thornicroft G (1995) Emergency psychiatric services in England and Wales. *BMJ.* **311**: 287–8.

13 Minghella E (1998) Home based emergency treatment. *Mental Health Pract.* **2**(1): 110–14.

14 Flowers K (1998) Intensive home treatment team: medication protocol and plan. *Mental Health Pract.* **1**(9): 24–7.

15 Shipman C, Dale J (1999) Responding to out-of-hours demand: the extent and nature of urgent need. *Family Pract.* **16**: 23–7.

16 Little GF, Watson DP (1996) The homeless in the emergency department: a patient profile. *J Accident Emerg Med.* **13**(6): 415–17.

17 Moore H, North C, Owens C (1997) Go home and rest? The use of an accident and emergency department by homeless people. *Emergency Nurse.* **5**(2): 28–31.

18 Pleace N, Quilgars D (1996) *Health and Homelessness in London. A Review.* King's Fund, London.

19 Hewett N (1998) In from the cold. *Health Service J.* **108**: 30–1.

20 Hutchinson K, Gutteridge B (1995) Health visiting homeless families: the role of the specialist health visitor. *Health Visitor.* **68**(9): 372–4.

21 Watt IS, Howell D, Lo L (1993) The health care experience and health behaviour of the Chinese: a survey based in Hull. *J Public Health Med.* **15**(2): 129–36.

22   Free C, White P, Shipman C, Dale J (1999) Access to and use of out of hours services by members of Vietnamese community groups in South London: a focus group study. *Family Pract.* (in press).

23   Leman P (1997) Interpreter use in an inner city accident and emergency department. *J Accident Emerg Med.* **14**(2): 98–100.

24   Boneham MA, Williams KE, Copeland JRM *et al.* (1997) Elderly people from ethnic minorities in Liverpool: mental illness, unmet need and barriers to service use. *Health Social Care Commun.* **5**(3): 173–80.

25   Tang M (1994) *Vietnamese Refugees: towards a healthy future. Final report: Vietnamese Health Project.* Save the Children/Deptford City Challenge/Optimum Health Services, London.

PART THREE

Future directions

Introduction

Previous sections have considered the purpose of out-of-hours care, the changing pattern of demand and service provision and the tensions between the expectations of the public and those of healthcare providers. The evidence base for out-of-hours care has been reviewed and examples of innovative services and models of good practice described.

In the final three chapters of this book we consider the future direction of out-of-hours primary care and its interface with 24-hour emergency care in more detail. Key themes of earlier chapters relating to quality and the integration of service provision are brought together. Drawing on the evidence presented in this book, we review the direction that developments in out-of-hours care are taking and address the question: what would make things work better?

CHAPTER TEN

The integration of services

Lesley Hallam

Chapter One highlighted the lack of co-ordination and communication between the different professionals and organisations involved in providing emergency, out-of-hours care within most European countries. It also demonstrated the diversity of the roles played by individual provider groups. Throughout successive chapters, lack of integration and the problems this creates have been a recurrent theme. The decision on which of a number of services is appropriate to their needs is frequently left to patients and their carers. Lacking medical skills and clear guidance, inevitably some make a choice which is considered inappropriate. The result is less than optimal care for the patient, frustration for patients and care providers and, not infrequently, an unnecessarily expensive episode of treatment for the health service.

Nonetheless, some heartening examples of changes in attitude and organisation have been highlighted. Chapter Five describes the way in which groups of GPs have come together to solve their common problems in providing an accessible and acceptable out-of-hours service whilst reducing the negative impact this has on the quality of their own personal and professional lives. Among the co-operatives they have formed, there are numerous examples of links being forged with other service providers. In providing accommodation and communication systems for community nurses, they are fostering a better understanding of the roles of each and creating opportunities to work together. Those who have chosen to locate their emergency centres within or adjacent to A&E departments have, at the least, demonstrated to hospital staff that it is not poor access to GP emergency services which brings primary care patients into hospital departments. In some instances, mutual respect for each other's problems has resulted in agreed guidelines on cross referrals. There are even examples of agreements on sharing reception and nurse triage staff.

Links between co-operatives and ambulance services are already strong in some areas, where ambulance service communication networks, vehicles and drivers are supplied, under contract, to local co-operatives. Less commonly, the introduction of evening and weekend pharmacy services in primary care emergency centres is being promoted.

Chapter Six describes how GPs have been successfully introduced on a sessional basis into hospital A&E departments, where they provide more appropriate, cost-effective services for primary care attenders than do SHOs. This has resulted in a greater understanding of each other's skills and knowledge and has opened the door for discussions on other joint approaches to treating patients out of hours. The example of the Croydon GP co-operative, which has contracted to treat up to 10 000 A&E 'primary care' consulters per annum, is one which could be taken up in other parts of the country, with mutual benefits for both groups.

Chapter Seven demonstrates the potential for nurse-led telephone triage systems. As the authors point out, the potential for a 'missed case' will remain whoever provides care but this has to be weighed against the merits of providing well-organised and much improved public access to medical information and advice. In Chapter Eight, the authors point out that one of the areas with most opportunity for co-ordination and integration is between minor injuries services and GP out-of-hours services. There is considerable potential for sharing premises and providing joint telephone answering and advice services staffed by experienced nurses.

Although the above examples demonstrate the advantages and possibilities of greater integration, Chapter Nine highlights the fact that there are some vulnerable groups of patients for whom a 'seamless' service is particularly important but difficult to achieve. Ensuring a high-quality service for the homeless, the mentally ill and the terminally ill is an important challenge for primary care groups in the future development of out-of-hours services.

Given that it is possible for different organisations to co-operate in providing an emergency service, it is worth considering why this does not happen to a greater extent.

A large part of the problem lies in deeprooted prejudices within different professional groupings. Individual services have developed in isolation, each with their own history and value systems. When these systems conflict or fail to reflect social changes, reform becomes an urgent priority. However, reforms commonly occur within individual services, often with little reference to their impact on other provider groups. Barriers to integration remain intact and may even be exacerbated. Of those countries surveyed in Chapter One, Denmark is a prime example of this. Despite sweeping reforms in the organisation of out-of-hours care provided by general practitioners, other services like A&E, dentistry, nursing, pharmacy and ambulances remained untouched. Patients unhappy with the reformed general practice system turn to A&E as an alternative. Whilst greater integration is now a priority, negotiations towards this end are proving slow and difficult.

Emergency care in the UK has its roots in historical differences between treatment for the wealthy and for the poor. The former had access to private physicians whose livelihood depended upon providing a high-quality personal service, in the patient's home if summoned. The latter relied on the charity of local hospital casualty departments. From the viewpoint of non-hospital physicians, hospital emergency departments were a form of competition, reducing their potential income by providing 'free' services to patients who might otherwise have paid to consult them. Even after the introduction of the GP 'panel' system, large groups within the population were not registered and continued to rely on hospital emergency care.

In the hospital system, prestige and rewards accrued to those doctors who were best insulated from the undifferentiated mass of patients. Clearly, 'casualty' doctors were least insulated. Accident and emergency became a Cinderella service, suffering from limited resources, poor facilities and an inability to attract the most able medical graduates. Improvements depended upon increasing the status of A&E as a specialty in its own right and hence in discouraging the attendance of patients with minor injuries and illnesses: the so-called 'primary care' patients. Meanwhile, extension of GP registration to all members of the population and the system of allowances and capitation fees which represented the bulk of GPs' income had changed GPs' attitudes to increased workload.

Rising demand for out-of-hours general practitioner services and rising attendances at A&E departments compounded the problem. Each provider group now feared that greater integration of services would lead to workload shifting. Each feared it would shift in their direction. Discussions surrounding the location of primary care emergency centres operated by GP co-operatives (*see* Chapter Five) reflect these fears.

> 'The fear of the [A&E department] consultant is that if a treatment centre is there for part of the time, it will attract primary care patients into the A&E department. And then, when the treatment centre is not running, his casualty officers will have to deal with the primary care cases.' (Co-operative founder member)

> 'The two things [A&E and GPs] have to be separate. It has to be independently financed and independently staffed. I do not subscribe to the idea of having GPs sitting in A&E so that everybody comes to A&E and GPs see the primary health care portion of it and we see the rest. I think it would bring confusion.' (A&E consultant)

Primary care attendances at A&E departments are often seen by staff as a failure on the part of the GP to provide an accessible service or to act as an adequate 'gatekeeper' to secondary care services rather than a conscious decision on the part of the patient to seek A&E care direct.

The increasing use of triage nurses in A&E departments, designed to ensure that high-priority patients with serious conditions receive rapid treatment, also ensures that patients with minor problems can face lengthy delays in crowded waiting rooms. The creation of regional major trauma centres, the closure of subsequently depleted small A&E departments and their replacement with local nurse-led minor injury units is intended to fulfil a number of purposes. The claim is that by creating a resource-rich environment able to deal cost effectively with larger numbers of seriously ill and injured patients, lives are saved. The specialty also gains in expertise and status, but patients with minor illnesses are constrained in their choice of care provider.

The role of community nursing was developed in isolation from that of general practice and with considerable distrust and hostility between the two groups. Local authorities were responsible for the provision of health visiting and district nursing services. These services were freely provided in clinics and in private homes. There were benefits from their uptake – free milk and simple remedies for childhood complaints, for instance. 'Family' doctors saw them as additional competition, taking potential fee-paying patients from their surgeries. Since the medical profession wielded considerable political power, demarcation laws were passed which confined local authority health workers to a purely advisory role. Pre-1948 GPs thus brought into the NHS an almost total lack of experience of working with other health professionals and a considerable degree of prejudice against them. District nurses concentrated their efforts mainly on visiting chronically ill patients discharged from hospital and patients referred by GPs directly to the local authority for injections, dressings and other treatment. Communication between the two groups remained poor.

When, in 1968, nursing, midwifery and health visiting workers became NHS employees and the move towards attachments to general practice and primary care teamwork began, this was resented and resisted by many within the community nursing professions. They had already experienced the devaluation of their skills and the restrictions imposed upon them by the demands of the medical profession. Assumptions about who should carry responsibility and authority and how demarcation lines should be drawn continue to haunt the NHS and influence current working relationships.

There is still only limited contact between general practitioners and community nurses outside normal surgery hours. However, some bridges are being built. The surgeries and health centres to which district nurses are attached during the daytime are normally closed out of hours, leaving them with no natural base and making them difficult to contact. There is growing recognition of the scope for general practitioner co-operatives to share their accommodation and communications equipment with district nursing teams.

The extent to which nurse practitioners, acting in triage and treatment roles, can be incorporated into a primary care out-of-hours service is the subject of considerable debate. As was pointed out in Chapter One, nursing input could reduce the workload of on-call general practitioners but would not necessarily reduce the amount of time they spend on call. Under current funding arrangements, in the majority of cases nurses' salaries would be met by the employing GPs. At the same time, their deployment would in all probability reduce GP income. If their salaries were met by the health service, they would undoubtedly prove more expensive than the GPs they replace. Furthermore, there are insufficient trained nurses within the workforce to fill new employment opportunities and difficulties in recruiting into the profession because of low levels of remuneration.

On a philosophical rather than a purely practical level, it could be argued that the employment of nurses out of hours is a further step in the direction of 24-hour access to primary care, rather than a 24-hour emergency service designed to provide immediate diagnosis and treatment for seriously ill patients. Many nurses would argue that it is not part of their role to diagnose illness, a continued acceptance of demarcation lines drawn long ago. There is also great controversy about their potential role in prescribing medication. Regardless of the specific tasks delegated to them by general practitioners, it is generally accepted that the patient's registered GP carries the legal responsibility for their actions.

Along with professional rivalries and differing perceptions of responsibilities and roles, one of the principal barriers to greater integration between services has been the separation of budgets. At the time of writing, the general medical services (GMS) budget funds general practitioner services; the hospital and community health services budget (HCHS) funds hospital, community nursing and ambulance services. Services which are hard pressed financially will naturally welcome opportunities to move costs to another's budget.

Services where there is a limited degree of integration suffer particular administrative and accounting problems. In community hospitals, for instance, patients who 'walk in' to a minor injuries or casualty facility are HCHS funded, although they may receive attention from the on-duty GP; patients who are asked by their GPs to attend the hospital out of hours for a primary care consultation are GMS funded. Distinguishing between the two can be problematic and is an unnecessary complication. The merger of these two funding streams in 1999 should provide greater opportunities for co-operation and integration, though again there may be conflicts if one group is seen to be taking an unfair share of what will then be a single cake.

As well as professional and financial barriers to integration, there are also difficulties with incompatible organisational systems, conflicting targets and guidelines and poor communication between services to be overcome.

Secondary care services and community nursing services are hierarchical and the staff within them are employed by their respective trusts. The roles and responsibilities of administrators, managers, clinicians and support staff are clearly defined. Each group has its own performance targets to reach and budgets are tightly controlled. General practitioners, together with community pharmacists and dentists, are independent contractors to the NHS. They are not subject to the same external controls (though there is a growing tendency to link their remuneration to specific performance targets). Persuading general practitioners to agree and work with each other towards common goals has been likened to 'herding cats'. The formation of GP co-operatives, described in Chapter Five, thus represents a major achievement. Nonetheless, the limited use and slow acceptance within co-operatives of protocols and guidelines is indicative of their highly individual nature. Where the two cultures meet, for instance in the attachment of community nurses to general practices, there is the potential for conflict and misunderstanding.

Despite the barriers between them, all these services share a common objective: to provide appropriate, effective and timely help for patients with medical needs. Greater integration and co-operation within and between the various provider groups is more likely to accomplish this than fragmented, unco-ordinated services which rely upon the judgement of the least experienced and most vulnerable member of the cast: the sick patient.

Whilst we have concentrated on GPs, nurses and A&E departments, there are many other health-related professional groups providing services out of hours. Attempts are being made to extend the role and improve patient awareness of the skills of community pharmacists. Their doors are frequently open in the evenings and at weekends, often as part of a local rota. Increasingly, 24-hour pharmacies operate in major population centres. In this, they are responding as much to commercial pressures as to the need to provide a service. Community pharmacists rarely operate as part of an emergency care network. Since on-call general practitioners carry a small stock of immediately necessary medications which can be used to provide emergency treatment until prescriptions can be filled, there is limited call for their services during the night.

Dentists too operate emergency rotas, but their services are little known by the general public. Further, dissatisfaction with remuneration levels in the NHS has led many dentists to concentrate on private practice, so that access to dentists for NHS patients has become a serious problem in many areas of the country. Patients with dental problems commonly contact their general practitioners. This too may be seen by GPs as an inappropriate use of services and increases professional tensions between GPs and dentists.

Ambulance services accept that theirs is a supporting role, but their expertise in control room operations, prioritisation and communications could be more widely deployed than is currently the case. In particular, the restrictions placed upon them in the disposition of patients mean that they are frequently the unwilling agents in delivering 'inappropriate' cases to A&E departments.

Clearly, there are numerous ways in which co-operation and collaboration between agencies are being explored and promoted. However, there is no 'master plan' for the future. Many of the innovations described have been led by general practitioners. This is hardly surprising, given that they have experienced the greatest impact from rising demand for out-of-hours care. However, they need not necessarily play the key role in controlling and co-ordinating an integrated primary care emergency service. With the development of primary care groups, GPs are more likely to become commissioners of emergency care, as well as providers. (Most fundholders in the past 'blocked back' to the health authorities that part of their budget which related to emergency care and so were not direct commissioners.) Whilst they may have local co-operatives they wish to commission, they will also have the opportunity to look to other organisations.

Community trusts have the potential to exploit the wide range of community nursing services which they provide, their existing links with GPs and other service providers and their clinical accommodation within communities. However, their current orientation is towards planned care rather than episodic emergency care outside normal surgery hours. They do not normally possess the sophisticated communications and record systems which would be necessary to support an integrated emergency service, though there is no reason why these could not be developed.

Acute hospital trusts with A&E facilities are experienced in providing emergency primary and secondary care, they have systems of nurse triage and prioritisation in place and some have experience in employing GPs to provide primary care in an A&E setting. Links are being established between GP co-operatives and A&E departments in some areas, with examples of shared personnel and agreements on cross referrals. Again, they do not possess the sophisticated communication systems needed, but these could be developed. The greatest drawback to co-ordinating services under a hospital system umbrella is likely to be cost. European healthcare systems which are orientated towards hospital-based services are generally more expensive than those based on primary care. There are also likely to be difficulties in persuading GPs that hospital co-ordination would not simply increase their workload exponentially, as hospitals 'unloaded' patients in their direction.

Commercial deputising services are in the business of providing out-of-hours care; they have sophisticated communications and record systems and a workforce of GPs already in place. They have existing links with GPs, knowledge of other sources of care, are developing telephone triage and increasingly provide primary care emergency centres, either alone or jointly with co-operatives. Whilst they currently operate largely in major population centres, their expansion into less well-populated areas is a possibility. The overwhelming problem is that they are 'for-profit' organisations with an interest in increasing demand rather than controlling it. They are unlikely to be acceptable to all other care providers.

The ambulance trusts also have the potential to develop into this role. They have the necessary communications and record systems, and existing links with GPs, community nursing staff and A&E departments. They employ and train paramedics and they are experienced in the prioritisation of calls. They are already playing a part in developing NHS Direct in some areas.

It should not be assumed that any particular provider organisation or professional group is best suited to be the main provider in all circumstances.

In the final chapter of this book, we draw together the lessons of preceding chapters to explore possible future directions in the provision of out-of-hours emergency care.

CHAPTER ELEVEN

Assuring quality

Jeremy Dale

'*Doing the right things, at the right time, for the right people, and doing them right – first time.*'[1]

Achieving quality in out-of-hours services involves managing the tension between demand (the public's perceptions about the *right time* to seek care), needs (commissioners' and providers' views about who are the *right people* to be utilising services) and resources (the *right things* that services should be capable of providing). It rests on making the most effective and efficient use of the available resources and technologies. Although some ways of delivering out-of-hours care do appear to be better than others, there is very little evidence that relates to the costs and quality of different models of out-of-hours and emergency care services or their applicability to particular settings. Consensus is lacking about what constitutes acceptable standards of out-of-hours care and the expectations of the public seem increasingly to be at odds with the views of the healthcare professions about the appropriate use of services. So, what then are the *right things* that out-of-hours services should be doing?

Quality has gained great emphasis in the agenda for the new NHS. The government has committed the NHS to ending fragmentation, unfairness, distortion, inefficiency and unacceptable variations in the quality of care (Box 11.1). A number of novel arrangements are being implemented. National service frameworks will describe how services can best be organised and the National Institute for Clinical Effectiveness (NICE) will provide clear guidelines about which treatments should be used for particular conditions. Clinical governance will bring greater accountability to each part of the NHS and all healthcare professionals will be involved (Box 11.2). The importance of including patients' views as part of a comprehensive assessment of quality of care is now enshrined in NHS policy. The National Survey of Patient and User

---

Box 11.1:   Six key principles underlying the new NHS

- To renew the NHS as a genuinely *national* service [with] ... fair access to consistently high-quality, prompt and accessible services right across the country.
- To make the delivery of healthcare against these new national standards a matter of *local* responsibility.
- To get the NHS to work in *partnership*. By breaking down organisational barriers and forging stronger links with local authorities, the needs of the patient will be put at the centre of the care process.
- To drive *efficiency* through a more rigorous approach to performance.
- To shift the focus onto quality of care so that *excellence* is guaranteed to all patients and quality becomes the driving force for decision making at every level of the service.
- To rebuild *public confidence* in the NHS as a public service, accountable to patients, open to the public and shaped by their views.

Experience will assess how well the NHS is delivering its services and whether local services are meeting patients' needs.

What impact will this have on out-of-hours services? What issues need to be considered in developing quality services? The challenge for those commissioning and delivering out-of-hours care is to apply what can be learnt from examples of good practice to their own local circumstances. In addition, those providing out-of-hours services will need to demonstrate their approach to managing the quality of their services. Primary care groups have considerable scope to influence the commissioning and provision of out-of-hours care and may be interested in developing and testing new models of organisation. NHS Direct could transform the ways in which patients access out-of-hours services and gain information and advice.

In this chapter, key issues relating to the quality of out-of-hours services are drawn together. These include identifying and understanding needs and demand, the availability and accessibility of services, the reliability and consistency of care, organisational and professional interfaces and patient acceptability.

Box 11.2: Main components of clinical governance

Clear lines of responsibility and accountability for the overall quality of clinical care
- A designated senior clinician responsible for ensuring that systems for clinical governance are in place and monitoring their continued effectiveness.
- Formal arrangements for managing clinical quality, perhaps through a clinical governance committee.
- Regular reports on the quality of clinical care given the same importance as monthly financial reports.
- An annual report on clinical governance.

A comprehensive programme of quality improvement activities which includes the following
- Full participation by all healthcare professionals in audit programmes.
- Evidence-based practice supported and applied routinely in everyday practice.
- Implementing the clinical standards of national service frameworks and NICE recommendations.
- Continuing professional development programmes to meet the development needs of individual health professionals and the service needs of the organisation.
- Appropriate safeguards to govern access to and storage of confidential patient information.
- Effective monitoring of clinical care with high-quality systems for clinical record keeping and the collection of relevant information.
- Processes for assuring the quality of clinical care is integrated with the quality programme for the organisation as a whole.

Clear policies aimed at managing risks
- Controls assurance which promotes self-assessment to identify and manage risks.
- Clinical risk systematically assessed with programmes in place to reduce risk.

Procedures to identify and remedy poor performance
- Critical incident reporting ensures that adverse events are identified and openly investigated, lessons are learned and promptly applied.
- Complaints procedures, accessible to patients and their families and fair to staff. Lessons are learned and recurrence of similar problems avoided.
- Professional performance procedures, which take effect at an early stage before patients are harmed and which help the individual to improve their performance whenever possible, are in place and understood by all staff.
- Staff supported in their duty to report any concerns about colleagues' professional conduct and performance. Clear procedures for reporting concerns so that early action can be taken to remedy the situation.

For the right people – the management of demand

There has been persistent controversy surrounding the demand for out-of-hours services. To what extent are the *right people* using out-of-hours services? Earlier chapters have considered the dramatic increase in demand for out-of-hours care which has occurred over the last few decades. There appears to have been a widening divergence between providers' views about appropriate service use and patterns of demand. This has been one of the principal impetuses for developing new service arrangements. Providers tend to view patients with clinical conditions that are already, or likely to become, urgent or life threatening as the *right people* to be making unplanned use of out-of-hours services.

Effective management of demand and expectations is required if services are to avoid becoming overburdened. But as we have seen, out-of-hours needs do not conform to a straightforward pattern. The difficulty both patients and clinicians face is being able to recognise urgency: the rare presentations that could become life threatening if care is delayed. For example, the headache that may be an early symptom of meningitis or a subarachnoid haemorrhage, the sore throat that might become a quinsy or acute epiglottitis or the abdominal pain that is due to appendicitis or a dissecting abdominal aortic aneurysm. Demand is influenced by a whole range of perceptions and beliefs about the incentives and disincentives of using the alternative help-seeking options recognised as being available. Erring on the side of caution inevitably leads to greater dependency on the health service and many people seeking advice or care for reassurance.

As the public's expectations of the health service grow and they become better informed and more aware of the potential risks associated with relatively minor symptoms, the threshold for seeking information and advice from a healthcare professional has fallen. Clinical and psychosocial needs are often inextricably linked, particularly during out-of-hours periods when social support systems may be less available. There is often a considerable overlay of anxiety and distress and for the clinician lacking information about the background and context of the patient, it may be difficult to appreciate the depths of their concerns. The relevance of existing communication and consultation skills training to the needs of out-of-hours care should be considered.

Attention is increasingly being focused on demand management strategies. Understanding demand and managing expectations are crucial if the goal of ensuring that the right people are treated by the right service at the right time is to be achieved. Expectations can be modified through the process of care, so influencing choice of subsequent care provider (*see*, for example, Chapter

Six). NHS Direct may have an important role to play in helping people swiftly to access care or information that is most relevant for their needs, regardless of their first point of contact with the health service (*see* Chapter Twelve). In addition to new structural arrangements like NHS Direct, new systems of training, professional development and public information will be required.

Doing it right – first time

Out-of-hours services, in common with much of the health service, have suffered from considerable variations in the quality and delivery of care. As we have seen, there have been inconsistencies in the availability, accessibility and organisation of services. There are differences in the patterns of treatment, referral decisions or self-care advice provided between individual healthcare professionals (such as variation in home-visiting rates between doctors working for the same out-of-hours service), between professional groups (such as between nurses and doctors giving telephone advice) and between provider organisations (such as between deputising services and co-operatives). These go beyond what can be explained by differences in the needs of individuals and populations. There are differences in the ways services are organised and structured, the ways patients are assessed and triaged and in response times.

There are considerable variations in the availability of out-of-hours services. Many areas, for example, lack out-of-hours community-based specialist help for palliative care or mental health problems, leading to needs not being met or being met inappropriately. Limited community psychiatric nurse availability out of hours, for example, may lead to avoidable admission for patients suffering from mental health problems who could otherwise have been maintained in the community. Lack of appropriately trained primary care professionals in A&E departments may result in unnecessary investigations, treatments and referrals. The limited availability of district nursing night cover in many areas may lead to increased GP contacts and avoidable acute or hospice admissions.

To what extent are services meeting the expectations of the public? The availability and accessibility of care are issues that are of particular concern to the public. Waiting times, for example, are a major cause of dissatisfaction with out-of-hours care, reflecting the anxiety, uncertainty, discomfort and inconvenience that patients and those caring for them experience. Effective management of patients' expectations might improve satisfaction with out-of-hours services. There is some evidence that patients who perceive waiting times to be shorter than anticipated express greater levels of satisfaction than those who perceive that they had waited longer. The extent to which patient satisfaction suffers because patients perceive services to be rushed or over-burdened is unclear. Increased waiting times are likely to be confounded by factors relating to the intensity of the service's workload and staffing levels, both of which may directly affect satisfaction. Providing information about waiting times, such as through NHS Direct, may help improve patient satisfaction with out-of-hours services.

Measuring and interpreting patients' satisfaction with health services is notoriously difficult given the tendency not to report dissatisfaction. Typically, at least 80% of respondents express satisfaction for any given question and many patients in the NHS appear reluctant to express critical comments. While to some extent satisfaction results from meeting or exceeding the patient's expectations about professional practice, professional behaviour and the organisation of care, the patient often lacks specific expectations against which to evaluate care.

Well-established methodologies for assessing satisfaction with out-of-hours general practice care are now available. In the early days of co-operatives, questionnaires were used that demonstrated very high levels of satisfaction. More sophisticated questionnaires[2] clearly demonstrate issues linked to dissatisfaction and are a suitable tool for monitoring patient satisfaction with out-of-hours GP services. Simplistic judgements about the acceptability of services based on unvalidated questionnaires need to be avoided.

Making the best use of resources – cost effectiveness

Ideally, the costs of out-of-hours care should be considered in terms of all the resources utilised in an episode of care (including whatever follow-up visits or referrals were involved). The start and endpoint for an episode of care may be difficult to determine and subsequent care may be provided by a range of different primary or secondary care services. Studies that look at resource use in the context of the volume and processes of care provided by a single service can be misleading unless seen within the context of other services being utilised by the population (e.g. within-hours care, A&E service use). From a societal perspective, cost effectiveness includes not only health service costs but also non-clinical costs (such as costs of transportation, time off work, childcare and other social costs incurred). By its very nature, out-of-hours care tends to be fragmented from care provided at other times.

There are several questions that remain about the organisation of out-of-hours services and their impact on quality and cost. For co-operatives, these relate to size, infrastructure, management, manpower planning and skill mix and triage and prioritisation systems. What, for instance, are the economies and diseconomies of scale associated with different sizes of co-op? What are the advantages and disadvantages of different types of setting for primary care emergency centres?

There is a need to strengthen the evidence base against which out-of-hours care can be judged. For many conditions, validated means of outcome measurement and guidelines or protocols are lacking against which out-of-hours care can be objectively judged. However, the inconsistencies observed in the process of care and its costs raise doubts about the validity and appropriateness of many therapeutic interventions and diagnostic decisions (including decisions about when a home visit is required, prescribing and referrals to specialist teams).

Improving quality

Features that support the delivery of high-quality services are well recognised (Box 11.3). Time will tell the extent to which the new quality agenda has an impact on the organisation and delivery of out-of-hours services. However, it seems inevitable that ever greater accountability will be required. Clinical governance is imposing a new framework for managing quality and organisations that take a proactive stance are likely to fare better. It should ensure that clear lines of accountability and responsibility for the overall clinical quality of services are established, with clear policies and procedures in place to manage risks and identify and remedy poor performance.

National agreement is needed on performance measures against which out-of-hours services can be judged. There is a need to encourage learning from experience and from other services. Professional and representative organisations like the Royal College of Nursing (RCN) and the National Association

---

Box 11.3:   Organisational and operational features of a quality service

- Explicit service aims and philosophy of care
- Shared commitment to the service goals
- Making the best use of available resources
- Clear roles and responsibilities
- Appropriate skill mix
- Commitment to ongoing training and professional development
- Adherence to agreed protocols, guidelines and standards
- Ongoing programme of quality assurance and clinical audit
- Co-ordination of services
- Involving users and public education
- Appropriate use of new technologies

of GP Co-operatives (NAGPC) may have an important role in disseminating models of good practice, including policies, procedures and guidelines. For example, a course focusing on communication skills during telephone consultation has been developed to meet GPs' learning needs and a manual for facilitators has been produced to enable the course to be delivered more widely.[3] The RCN (1998) has recently published guidance for best practice in nurse telephone consultation[4] and the NAGPC[5] has produced guidance on the employment of nurses within co-operatives.

Quality improvement needs to be an ongoing process and audit, professional development and other components of organisational learning are all important components. Strategies to improve quality need to be linked to research and evaluation; as we have seen, there is a need to strengthen the evidence base in relation to out-of-hours care.

More sophisticated planning of out-of-hours services is needed to manage quality within the context of the general shift towards a more '24-hour' society. To date, the public and patients have been minimally involved in the planning of new out-of-hours service developments and often lack information about new arrangements. This relates particularly to the development of co-operatives, with increasing reliance on telephone advice and the shift away from home visiting. As we have seen, demand reflects complex inter-relationships between perceptions of need, health beliefs, understanding and expectations of the healthcare system. It is often influenced by advice from family, friends, neighbours or other lay informants and an appraisal of what might be the social costs incurred by different actions, such as the impact of taking time off work or needing to arrange care for other dependants. Simplistic messages are unlikely to have much impact on the public's use of services.

It is clearly important that consistent, appropriate and comprehensible advice and information are targeted to the public to help people self-care and make more appropriate use of services. In addition to NHS Direct, the publication and distribution of locally relevant advice and information booklets may be helpful together with innovative use of the Internet.

A number of concerns have been identified in earlier chapters in relation to the equity of services. The extent of specialist service provision, for example for mental health and palliative care needs, is unknown on a national scale. There is evidence that some people, such as those lacking private transport, those with dependants, those lacking social networks and support or those with language differences, have been disadvantaged by the shift from home visiting to telephone advice and base consultations. This may lead to greater use of the ambulance service and A&E departments rather than out-of-hours GP services. Certain groups may have difficulties in communicating out-of-hours needs over the phone, for example people with learning difficulties or language differences. There is a need to consider the provision of such interventions as patient transport and interpretation services to ensure equity of access to services.

Finally, quality improvement needs to occur in the context of the whole urgent-care system. Out-of-hours care involves a multiplicity of interfaces between different health service organisations, professional groups and within-hours services. At each interface, communication and the continuity of care can easily break down. There are many issues that need to be addressed relating to the use of IT and decision support and information sharing. Shared procedures and policies and compatible methods of data recording and use of IT may all help to maintain continuity. However, lack of knowledge and understanding between agencies about each other's services is the first barrier that needs to be overcome before such developments can occur. These issues are discussed further in Chapters Ten and Twelve.

References

1   Department of Health (1997) *The New NHS: modern, dependable.* HMSO, London.

2   McKinley JK, Manku-Scott T, Hastings AM, French DP, Baker R (1997) Reliability and validity of a new measure of patient satisfaction with out of hours primary medical care in the United Kingdon: development of a patient questionnaire. *BMJ.* **314**: 193–8.

3   Jessop J, Armstrong E, Foster J, Aukland R (1998) *Conducting Telephone Consultations: a two day experiential course for GPs. Facilitators pack.* Lambeth, Southwark and Lewisham Out of Hours Project, King's College School of Medicine and Dentistry, London.

4   Royal College of Nursing (1998) *Nurse Telephone Consultation: information and good practice.* RCN, London.

5   National Association of GP Co-operatives (1998) *The Role of Nursing in Co-operatives.* NAGPC, London.

CHAPTER TWELVE

A vision for the future

Chris Salisbury

Themes

Throughout this book a number of themes have been apparent. In this final chapter we will review some of these themes and their likely impact on the future planning of out-of-hours general practice services. The wider implications for primary care will be considered and we will describe one model of organisation which may offer a way forward.

The first theme is the way in which the organisation of out-of-hours services has rapidly evolved. As provider organisations responded to changing patient demand, changes in service in turn led to further modification in patients' expectations. This iterative process is also reflected in the expectations of doctors and other healthcare professionals, as we shall see below.

New forms of service development

The most important development has been the rapid growth in the number of general practitioners choosing to work in large co-operatives. Many of these co-operatives have invested heavily in buildings, communication systems and organisational systems to provide a service which may be more responsive, better organised and better equipped than the surgeries in which the member GPs work in the daytime. This is having an impact on the type of service that patients expect. In the past many patients may have felt reluctant to 'bother' their doctor outside surgery hours, knowing that he or she might be relaxing or asleep in bed. Although doctors complain that out-of-hours calls are frequently about trivial problems, many people are still reluctant to contact a doctor, particularly at night, when perhaps they should. As patients perceive that doctors are working in 'shifts' and as they become used to relating to large impersonal organisations rather than the domestic scale of their local general practitioner on call from home, this reluctance may dissipate.

Just as patients' expectations and behaviour may alter in response to their experience of new out-of-hours arrangements, so might the attitudes of general practitioners. Continuity of care has been considered one of the core values in the ideology of general practice. Until recently, this has been interpreted as requiring doctors to be personally available outside surgery hours or to work in a rota within the practice. This interpretation was increasingly challenged during the early 1990s. A number of authors stressed the importance of doctors accepting their own limitations, adopting non-paternalistic relationships with patients which were not based on the myth of the doctor as superhuman and indispensable.[1] With the growth of co-operatives, this process of challenging notions about core values in general practice may have accelerated. Doctors increasingly see medicine as a job like any other, with clearly defined working and off-duty hours. Some general practitioners have described how the use of co-operatives has given them uninterrupted leisure time and has enabled them to rediscover non-medical pursuits.[2–4]

'I have worked two sessions for our co-op each month. I've seen as many patients out-of-hours in these two sessions as I would have with my one-in-four rota. And I have my life back, my family have me back and, I hope, my patients have their doctor back.'[2]

'(The co-operative has ...) dramatically improved my lifestyle. Even the cat seems happier and the garden certainly looks better.'[3]

'I hated it (being on call). It was really colouring what I did in the day as well ... I found it an enormous intrusion on my privacy when the calls came into the house ... and I actually behaved quite out of character. I often could be quite off-hand to the patients. I'm not really like that and I used to hate myself. It was only when speaking to one or two other doctors that I realised that I was not alone ... that the other doctors behaved irrationally.' (Quote from unpublished interviews with GPs by Lesley Hallam)

Even though the number of overnight shifts carried out by doctors in a co-operative system may be greatly reduced compared with their previous commitments, some co-operatives have described how doctors increasingly resent the shifts they still have to work and high rates of pay have to be offered to attract doctors to work at unsocial hours, particularly overnight.

Integration

The second recurring theme is the importance of integration. As large organisations such as co-operatives have grown in importance, it has been increasingly important to consider how the various providers of out-of-hours care can work together to provide comprehensive and 'seamless' help and to avoid duplication. Some of the advantages and difficulties involved in the integration of services have been discussed in Chapter Ten. Although there are substantial problems relating to funding, confidentiality, incompatibility of organisational systems and differences in professional responsibilities, a trend towards increased integration of services seems inevitable. In particular, an integrated service should make it possible to more accurately match professional skills to patients' needs. At present, different patients with identical problems may receive very different responses according to whether they contact a GP or an A&E department or dial 999 for an ambulance. An appropriately organised service would provide a consistently high quality of care, as discussed in Chapter Eleven, irrespective of the patient's route of entry to the health system.

Skill mix

A third theme is that of skill mix and the involvement of a wider range of professionals. At present, doctors provide most out-of-hours care, although they may not be the most appropriate people to deal with many of the problems that patients present. A more integrated service may need a different balance of professional skills and would probably require a larger number of nurses and healthcare assistants than are currently employed, with fewer doctors. There is also potential for a much greater role for local pharmacies in providing advice and treatment for the common minor ailments which make up a large proportion of out-of-hours calls.

The involvement of nurses in providing telephone advice and triage has been discussed in preceding chapters. If nurses and others are going to take on a substantial proportion of the out-of-hours workload, this will have implications for their training programmes. There may also be recruitment difficulties, as it is doubtful whether there will be a sufficient number of nurses or pharmacists willing to work at unsocial times. The obvious means of overcoming this problem is through premium rates of pay, but this may lead to a more expensive system. The cost effectiveness of different models of care will need careful investigation. The complexities of the payment system for GPs and the lack of explicit costing for their out-of-hours work means that there are a variety of ways of costing the present GP-based system. This makes it difficult to compare the cost effectiveness of new models of care.

Demand management

A fourth theme is the management of demand. We have seen in Chapter Two that there appears to be considerable variability between different areas in the demand for out-of-hours care, but that overall rates of demand appear to have increased. It is likely that if services are more convenient, more accessible and provide a higher quality of service, then demand will continue to rise. It will be important to consider how this demand should be managed.

The rise in demand has occurred in the context of a consumerist approach to healthcare, but it is unlikely that any state-funded service will be able to meet a demand for instantly accessible help, 24 hours a day. A limited campaign of patient education has been initiated, but this is based on the somewhat patronising assumption that if patients were better informed they would not call in the out-of-hours period. Patients may (and do) argue that the problem does not lie with their level of knowledge but with the way that services are organised. Since they pay for the service through their taxes, they can reasonably expect that help will be available when they feel they need it. No amount of patient education will remove this conflict of interest between the convenience of patients and health professionals. If people find it inconvenient to contact a healthcare professional in the daytime and if similar services are available in the evening, it is a perfectly rational response to attempt to arrange an evening consultation. The management of demand is therefore likely to be a continuing challenge. This will require more explicit acknowledgement that 24-hour routine primary healthcare is unaffordable, better systems for categorising and prioritising calls, and better integration with routine services to enable callers to access convenient care in the daytime.

Implications for general practice

The growth of large organisations such as GP co-operatives has implications for the future of general practice as a whole. Co-operatives in many ways represent a further step in a long-term trend towards GPs working in larger and larger groups. This started with the move from single-handed practices into partnerships and is evident in the increasing average size of these partnerships. The success of co-operatives in demonstrating the value of practices working together is one of the factors which may have encouraged the idea of primary care groups as a model for purchasing all healthcare. Many of these groups have been built on relationships between practices which were established through doctors working together in out-of-hours co-operatives.

As organisations become larger and less based on local practices and local communities, they become less personal. The decreasing importance of personal continuity of care and the separation between daytime practice-based care and out-of-hours care call into question some of the assumptions about how general practice should be organised. For example, it could be argued that there is now no need for people to register with a doctor near their home. Many people, particularly those who commute, may find it more convenient to see a doctor near their place of work. Just as car owners have regular contact with a local garage but may also belong to a national break-down service, it is conceivable that patients could register for daytime primary care in one area, knowing that they had access to an alternative impersonal but efficient system for primary care in the evenings and at weekends.

As well as challenging the importance of continuity, one of the core values of general practice, the success of co-operatives in enabling large groups of doctors to work together has encouraged them to expand their activities beyond out-of-hours care. One co-operative, for example, has set up a locum agency and another has created an Internet web page offering advice about minor illness. As co-operatives have gained experience in efficient call management, telephone triage and rapid treatment for acute medical problems, some have begun to provide similar services in the daytime. This represents a predictable next step in the depersonalisation of general practice, with patients relating to an organisation rather than any individual doctor. Co-operatives, possibly run by PCGs, could progressively take over the management of acute primary care needs. They could provide telephone advice and see patients requiring a same-day consultation, leaving non-urgent pre-booked care as the responsibility of the member practices. Some patients would probably find this idea very welcome. Other groups of patients, such as the psychologically needy and those with young children, receive a large proportion of their care on a same-day basis and for these patients the co-operative could become their main medical provider. The possible detrimental effects on the care available to these groups of patients should be carefully considered.

The development of large centralised services can be seen as a response to changing patient demand and changes in the medical workforce, as discussed in Chapters One and Two. A further driver for change has been developments in communications technology. In the same way that computers have revolutionised many commercial activities, such as banking, by making it possible to work in new ways, so technology has been a powerful influence on how out-of-hours care is provided. This process can be traced back to the invention of telephones and then radio-pagers (or 'bleeps'). The increased accessibility of doctors led to changing expectations about their availability and speed of response. Many out-of-hours providers now have computerised call management systems and computer-driven protocols for care, enabling them to cope with a large volume of calls. Some have sophisticated ways of keeping in touch with multiple sites through mobile facsimile systems and of keeping track of their vehicles through satellite technology. The possibilities offered by improved communications technology will continue to challenge our assumptions about the best way to deliver care and will make possible levels of integration which could not have been previously achieved.

In Chapter One we suggested that there were three fundamental questions which needed to be addressed in order to reform out-of-hours care in the UK. We asked whether the interests of consumers or professionals were paramount; whether the system should seek to provide 24-hour care or emergency care only; and whether services should be the responsibility of individual providers or organised at a regional or national level. It now seems clear that a new balance is needed between patients and providers. The rampant consumerism of the 1980s no longer appears sustainable or affordable within the health service, but professionals cannot continue to arrange services to meet their own convenience, on the assumption that patients will be grateful for what they are given. The future organisation of out-of-hours care requires a model which meets patients' essential medical needs at affordable cost. Such a model of care is likely to rely on the use of a wider and more appropriate range of professional skills, with better integration and less duplication of services, facilitated by technological advances.

A proposed model for the future

What would an 'ideal' system for out-of-hours care therefore look like? It has been suggested that a successful system is one that:

- provides high-quality care for urgent medical problems
- is satisfactory in the eyes of patients
- provides doctors with reasonable working hours and conditions
- supports rather than detracts from daytime primary care
- is provided at an affordable cost.

How might one design a model of care which achieves all five aims? A logical first step would be a single point of access for all out-of-hours medical care. By the end of the year 2000, NHS Direct helplines will be available to the entire population of England (*see* Chapter Three). At present, NHS Direct provides an alternative source of assistance to that offered by existing providers. However, NHS Direct could become the *only* way into the system. This would be convenient for patients and would also be an effective way of managing demand. The present system is inconsistent, does not necessarily steer patients to the best form of help and provides much duplication of effort, but there remain many gaps in services. For example, it is ironic that most primary care centres have a policy of restricting access to those who have first been assessed on the telephone, yet patients with similar primary care problems can walk into an A&E department (intended to cope with more serious medical emergencies), often next door to the primary care centre.

The solution would be to view A&E departments as one specialist component in an integrated system. Access would only be possible following an initial telephone assessment or by ambulance (although access to an ambulance would also have been initially through an integrated call centre). Patients without telephones who arrive unexpectedly at A&E would be triaged at the door, as happens now, but would be redirected to a primary care centre unless their problem required specialist attention.

Although restricting open access to A&E departments might be politically difficult, this would offer improvements for patients in terms of obtaining high-quality care in the most appropriate environment. Such a strategy would require a sustained marketing approach to persuade people of the advantages to be gained. Safeguards would be needed to ensure that those with special needs were not disadvantaged (*see* Chapter Nine).

All calls, whether requiring telephone advice, a consultation with a doctor, attendance at A&E following a minor accident or an ambulance in a medical emergency, would be made to the same number. Call management would be handled at regional centres, which would be linked electronically to local provider units. The range of providers of help would be wide, including A&E departments, ambulance stations, primary care centres staffed by general practitioners, community nurses, 24-hour pharmacies, social services (particularly for rapid-response home support), and community mental health teams. Telephone calls would be answered rapidly, because of the need to respond to medical emergencies, but callers requiring less urgent advice may have to be queued or telephoned back at times of high demand.

The call management centre would hold a current database of NHS information. This could include patients' registration details, along with their previous medical history, current medication and details of any allergies. One of the claimed disadvantages of care from co-operatives and deputising services is that the consulting doctor does not have access to the patients' medical records. However, using technology in this way will make it possible for various providers to share information, which is available at any time and at a number of sites. A doctor or nurse could therefore know a substantial amount about a patient, even if they did not know them personally. This process could also be used to increase efficiency and to reduce the flow of paper. Following an encounter, details of the consultation could be sent electronically to the patient's registered GP and automatically filed in the patient's computerised medical record. This system is in accord with the information strategy for the NHS, which anticipates that all computerised general practices will be connected to NHSnet (a secure information network for the health service) by the end of 1999 and that electronic health records allowing 24-hour access to patients' medical details will be developed in the longer term (within 4–6 years).

Although technically feasible, these developments require far greater stand-ardisation of data entry and coding than currently exist and raise important questions about the confidentiality of information. One solution may be for local doctors and nurses to 'opt in' further information when they felt it should be made available about individual patients (for example, those who were terminally ill). Details about particular patients would be logged with the central database, rather than the out-of-hours service having access to information about all patients.

At the regional call management centre the trained operator would make an initial assessment of the urgency of the caller's problem, following proto-cols developed with the various providers of care. Details of patients with medical emergencies would be transferred electronically to local ambulance stations for them to respond. Patients needing less urgent advice or a more detailed assessment on the telephone would be transferred to a nurse, who would manage the call along the lines discussed in Chapter Seven of this book. Following a nurse assessment, some patients would need a face-to-face consultation. The nurse would be able to book an appointment at a primary care centre or a home visit and could direct the patient to one of the local primary care centres or if necessary arrange transport.

Regional call centres might cover an area the size of a county or several adjoining counties, but primary care centres would be situated in local cen-tres of population so that they are easily accessible. The exact arrangement of centres would depend on local circumstances, particularly the population density of an area. Many centres may be placed adjoining A&E departments. Doctors and nurses carrying out home visits would be based at these local primary care centres. In this way, they could provide a reasonably rapid response and there could also be flexibility for staff to work in the primary care centre when they are not needed on home visits.

The above model has much in common with the Danish system of out-of-hours care, which was reformed in 1992 to address the same problems as have been experienced in the UK. Following the reforms, the proportion of out-of-hours callers receiving home visits dropped by more than half (from 46% in 1990 to 18% in 1996), with the proportion of patients receiving tele-phone advice and attending a centre increasing to 48% and 33% respectively. The system has proved popular with doctors and has fulfilled its aims. Although there was an initial drop in patient satisfaction, this is now returning to former levels.[5]

In order to develop such a model of out-of-hours care, several important obstacles would need to be overcome. As described in Chapter Ten and earlier in this chapter, these obstacles include interprofessional rivalries, medicolegal responsibilities, technical difficulties and conflicts generated by providers being funded from different budgets.

The effect on the future of primary care

The model described above suggests the next step in a process which has been evolving rapidly over the last decade. Will this model be 'the answer' to the problem of out-of-hours care and will the pace of change then slacken?

The developments in out-of-hours primary care in the early 1990s were made possible by a number of contractual changes in general practice. These changes were introduced because of widespread resentment amongst general practitioners, with many doctors demanding to withdraw from providing out-of-hours work altogether. The efficiencies offered by working together in large organisations such as co-operatives may have provided doctors with a 'breathing space', enabling them to cope with a greater demand for care. However, it is predictable that within a few years, general practitioners will again be demanding a separation between daytime and out-of-hours work. This will have been fuelled by a continuing increase in patient demand, the increased depersonalisation of doctor–patient relationships and the proven viability and acceptability of a comprehensive integrated 24-hour primary healthcare service. The issue of a global 24-hour general practice contract will have become irrelevant.

Writing in 1997, in conclusion to a book about the history of general practice in the NHS, John Horder (past president of the Royal College of General Practitioners) stated that:

> 'erosion of the tradition of personal care is now a real danger, and its preser-vation is one of the great challenges we face in these times of uncertainty and confusion over the future direction of the NHS and of general practice within it.'[6]

These sentiments echo those voiced by Iona Heath and many others who have sought to defend traditional notions of primary care. Heath expresses in dramatic fashion the choices which face the public and the medical profession.

> 'If patients and citizens want – and increasingly demand – a high-quality, consumer-orientated service with the full range of primary care available around the clock then a new general practice contract will be needed. The work-ing day and out-of-hours components will have to be contracted for separately

and many more members of primary care teams will have to be available out of hours. Such changes could have enormous consequences, with the possibility that general practice will be fragmented, privatised and changed fundamentally.'[7]

Although out-of-hours care represents only a small proportion of all primary care workload, it is the point at which the tensions between patients and professional expectations are felt most acutely. The challenges and difficulties have led to a period of intense innovation and experimentation. These developments may prove influential well beyond out-of-hours care, leading to a re-evaluation of core values in general practice, changes in relationships between local practices, the reconsideration of the place of a GP as an independent contractor in an integrated health service and, most importantly, a change in the nature of the relationship between patients and their doctors.

References

1   Iliffe S, Haug U (1991) Out of hours work in general practice *BMJ.* **302**: 1584–6.

2   Bates B (1997) Out-of-hours co-op gave back my life. *Pulse.* **October 18**: 51.

3   Carlowe J (1997) Growth of co-ops has lifted a huge burden from GPs. *Pulse.* **May 17**: 2–3.

4   Anon (1997) Co-ops are main morale booster. *Pulse.* **June 7**: 2–3.

5   Christensen MB, Olesen F (1998) Out of hours service in Denmark: evaluation five years after reform. *BMJ.* **316**: 1502–5.

6   Loudon I, Horder J, Webster C (1998) *General Practice under the National Health Service 1948–1997.* OUP, Oxford.

7   Heath I (1995) General practice at night. *BMJ.* **311**: 466.

Index